Aortic Stenosis - Current Perspectives

Edited by Peter Magnusson

Published in London, United Kingdom

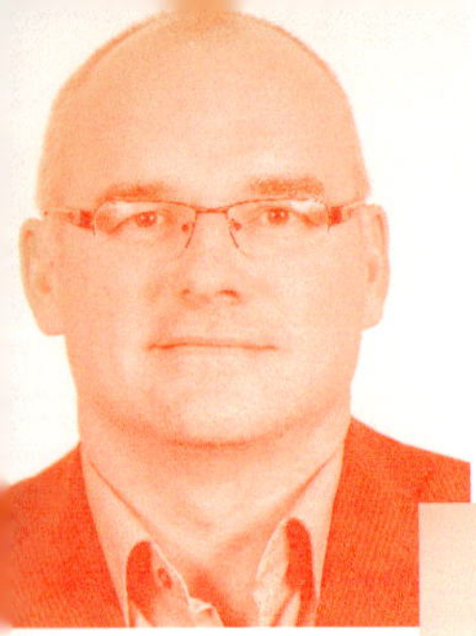
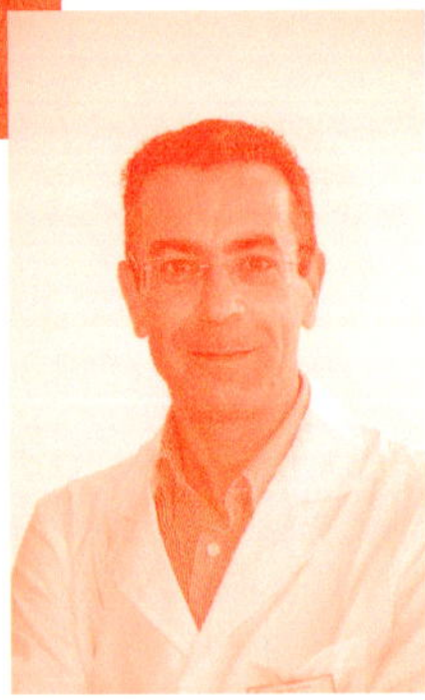
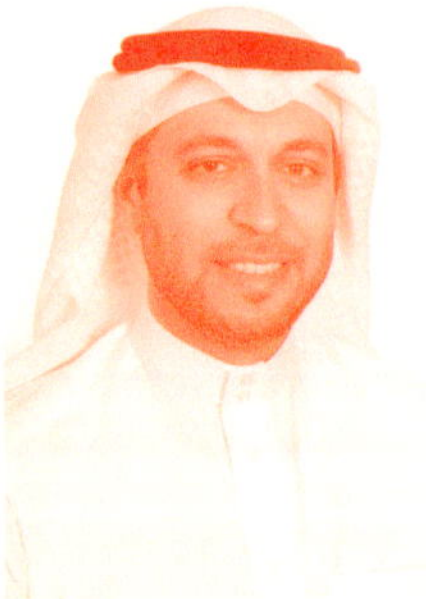
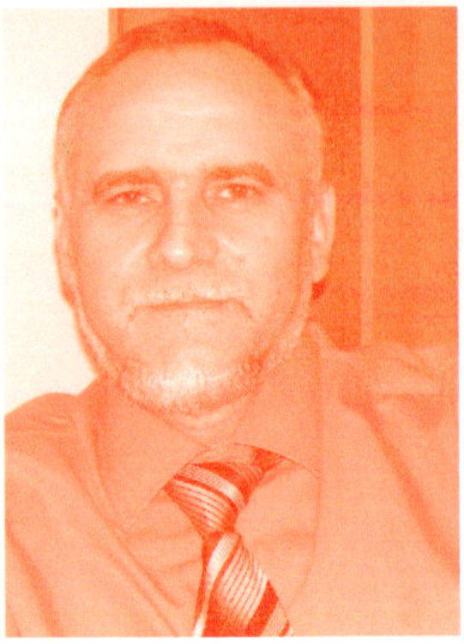
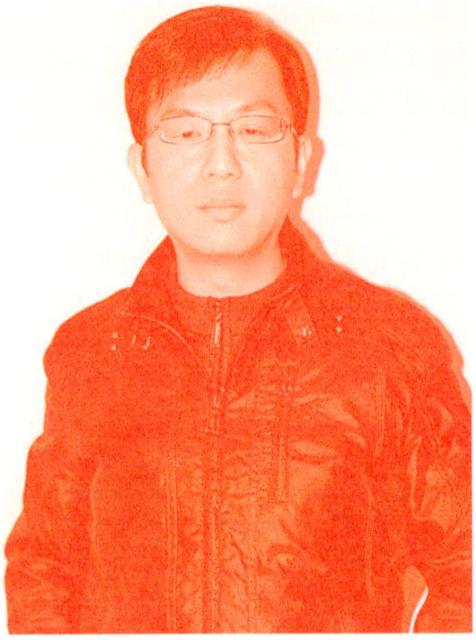
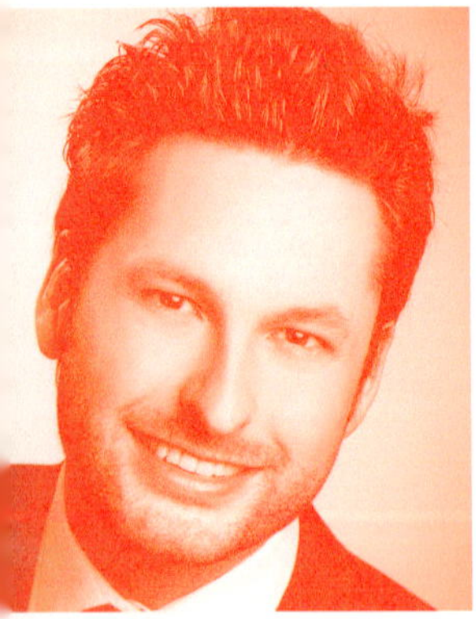
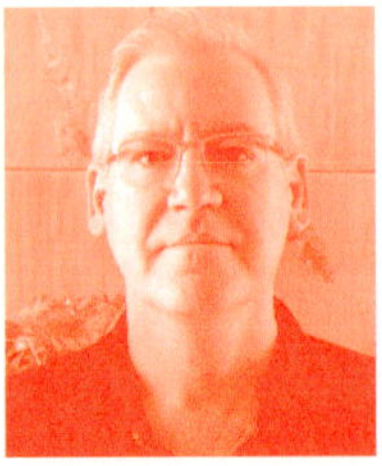

IntechOpen

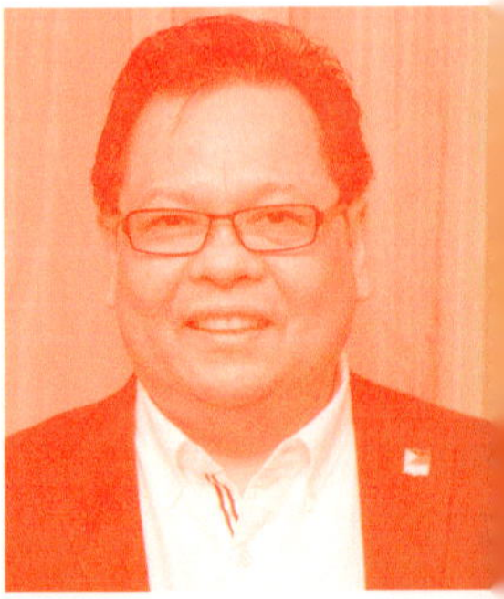
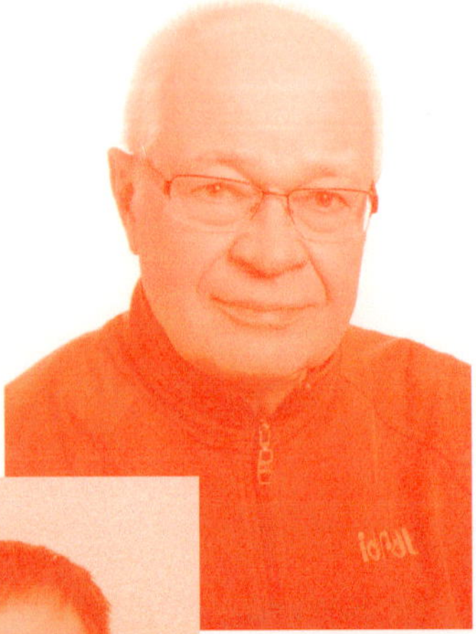
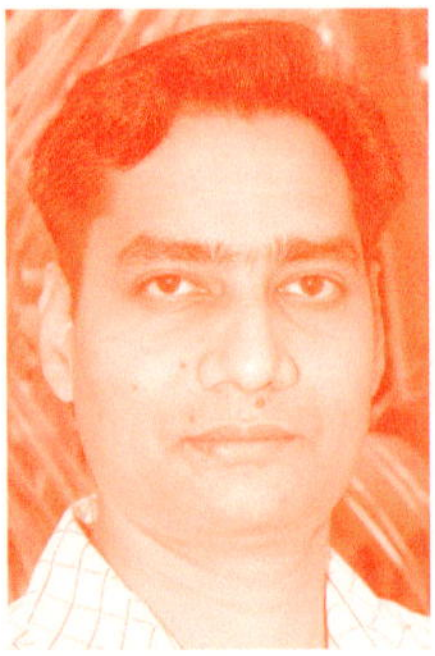
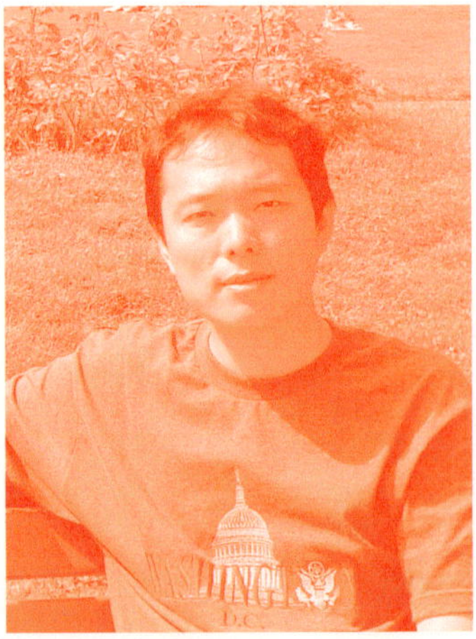
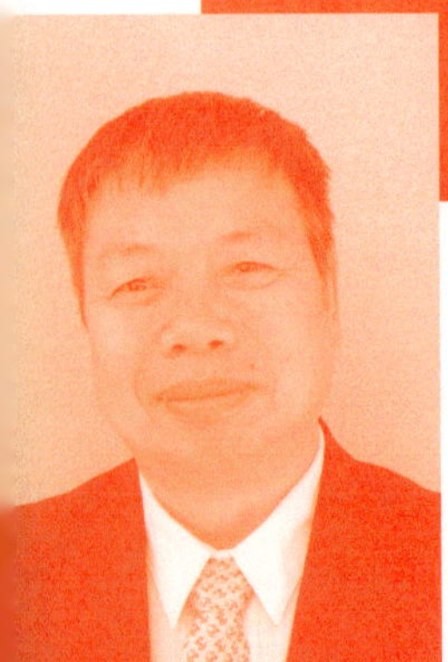
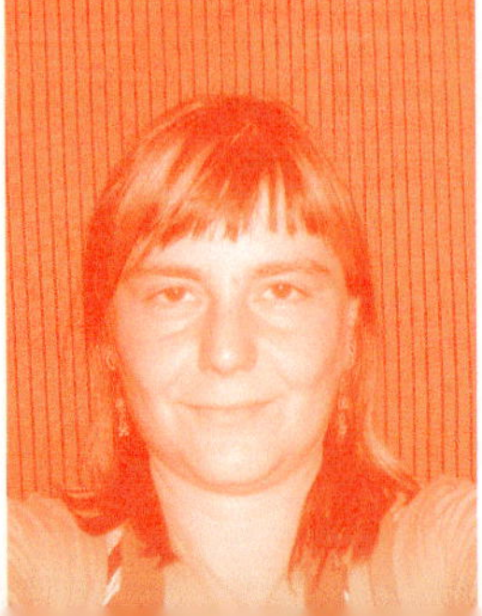

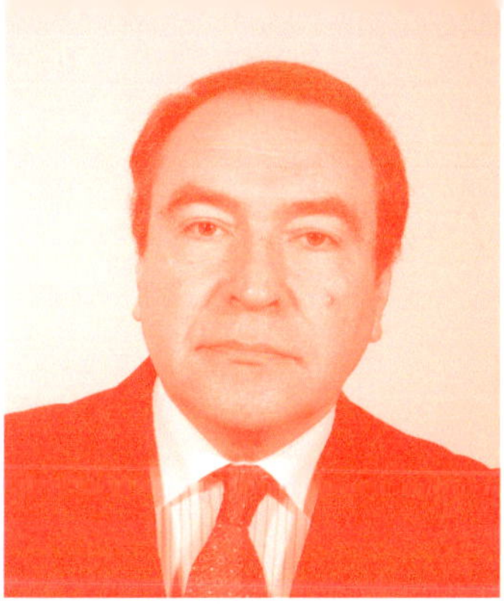
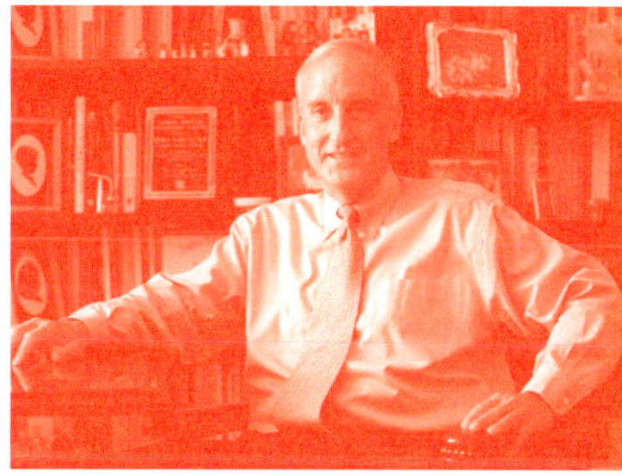
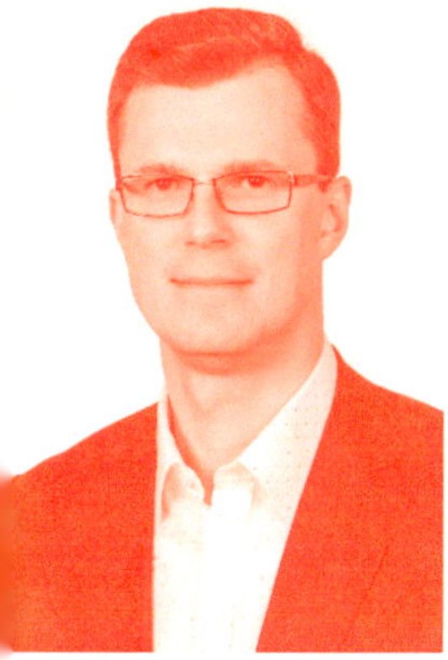
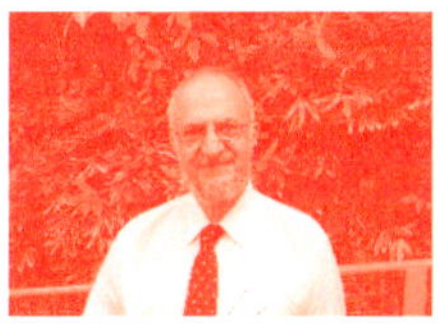
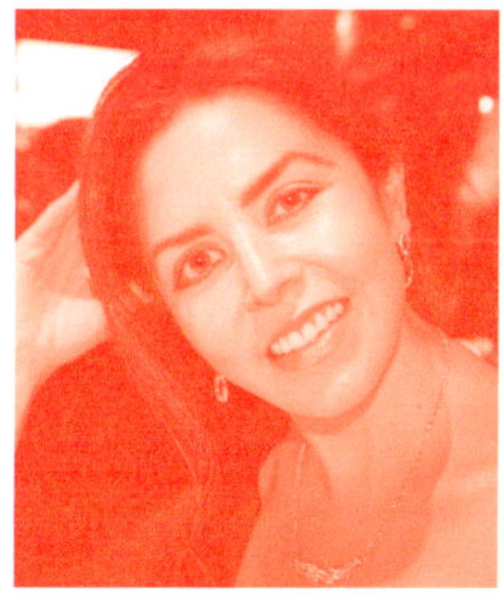

Supporting open minds since 2005

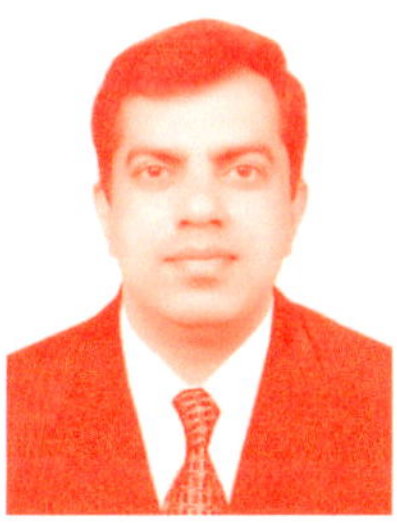
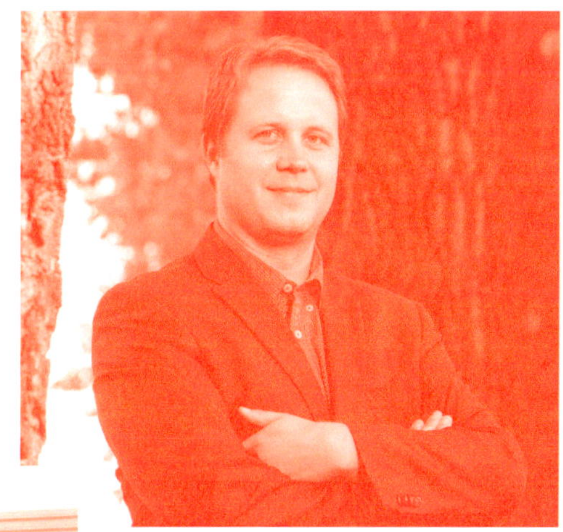
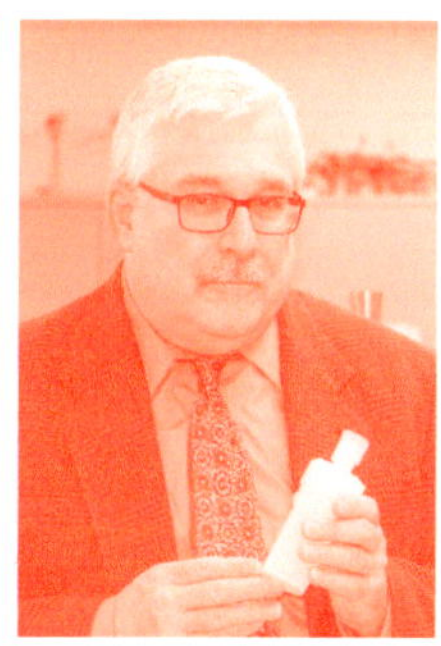
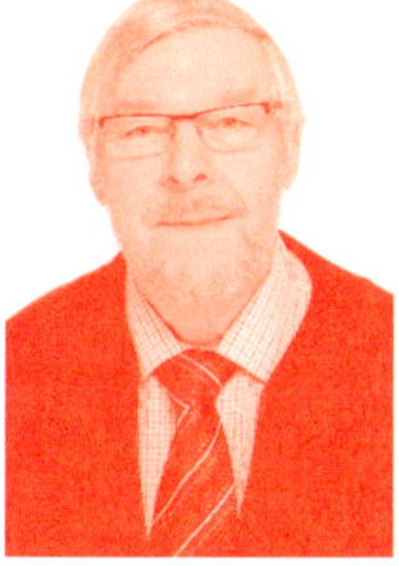
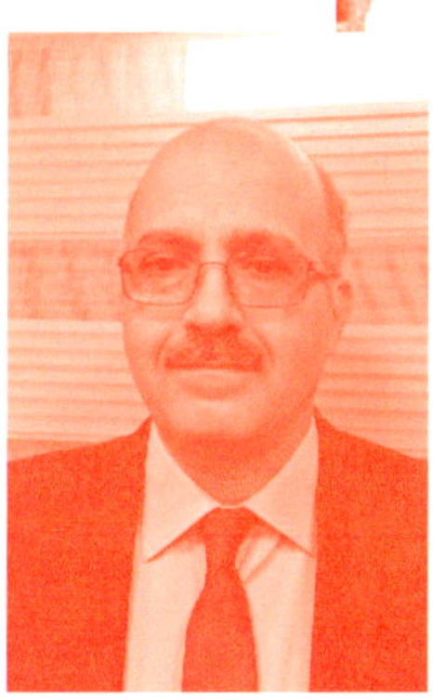
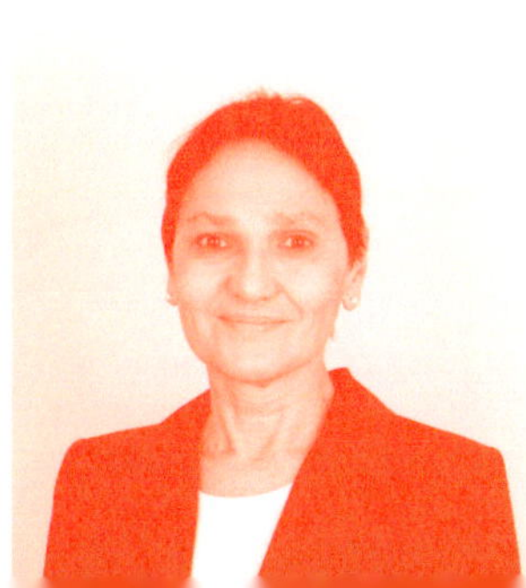
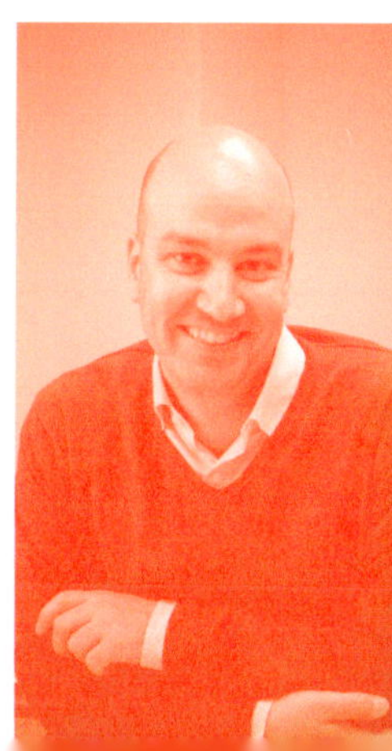

Aortic Stenosis - Current Perspectives
http://dx.doi.org/10.5772/intechopen.78174
Edited by Peter Magnusson

Contributors
Aleksandra Domanjko Petrič, Anja Perovič, Tanja Švara, Peter Dovč, Naresh Kumar Monigari, Anoop Agarwal, Omer Leal, Diego Sanchez-Valenzuela, Juan Bustamante-Munguira, Eva Maria Aguilar Blanco, Angels Figuerola-Tejerina, Rajesh Nair, Faeez Mohamad Ali, Vindhya Wilson, Susan Kwon, Aasha Gopal, Peter Magnusson

First published in London, United Kingdom, 2019 by IntechOpen
IntechOpen is the global imprint of INTECHOPEN LIMITED, registered in England and Wales, registration number: 11086078, The Shard, 25th floor, 32 London Bridge Street
London, SE19SG - United Kingdom
Printed in Croatia

British Library Cataloguing-in-Publication Data
A catalogue record for this book is available from the British Library

Additional hard and PDF copies can be obtained from orders@intechopen.com

Aortic Stenosis - Current Perspectives
Edited by Peter Magnusson
p. cm.
Print ISBN 978-1-78923-851-8
Online ISBN 978-1-78923-852-5
eBook (PDF) ISBN 978-1-83962-232-8

For EU product safety concerns:
IN TECH d.o.o., Prolaz Marije Krucifikse Kozulić 3, 51000 Rijeka, Croatia, info@intechopen.com or visit our website at intechopen.com.

Meet the editor

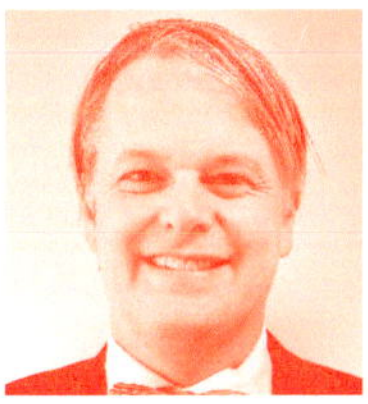

Peter Magnusson is a senior consultant in cardiology and active in research projects in arrhythmia, cardiomyopathy, heart failure, and valvular disease. He is affiliated with the Karolinska Institute, Sweden, and the Center for Research and Development, Gävleborg, at Uppsala University, Sweden. Dr. Magnusson's research involves epidemiological studies, qualitative methods, observational studies, and randomized controlled trials. He is passionate about teaching and supervision, especially in academic projects. Currently, he is striving for implementation of research findings in the healthcare system.

Contents

Preface

Aortic stenosis is the most frequent reason for valvular intervention, and due to an ageing population its incidence is likely to increase. As such, healthcare providers need to be aware of the condition and possess basic knowledge of how to manage it. Echocardiographic assessment of left ventricular outflow gradient and aortic valve area is fundamental for classifying severity of the stenosis. Historically, a surgical approach has been primarily used for treatment, however, a catheter-based approach has emerged as a preferable alternative in many patient subgroups, including those at intermediate and low levels of risk. This book covers diverse aspects of the etiology, diagnosis, treatment, and follow-up of patients with aortic stenosis.

Peter Magnusson
Karolinska Institute,
Sweden

Chapter 1

Introductory Chapter: Aortic Stenosis

Peter Magnusson

1. Definition and symptoms

Aortic stenosis is the most frequent cause of valvular intervention in the Western world and is increasing with age. Thus, awareness and basic knowledge about the management of aortic stenosis are important for a diverse spectrum of health-care providers. When a diagnosis of aortic stenosis is established, careful attention and management are warranted by several health-care providers including general practitioners, internists, geriatricians, anesthesiologists, thoracic surgeons, and imaging experts, besides cardiologists.

Symptoms of aortic stenosis are unspecific and often vague as the disease progression is typically slow. However, when patients finally present with symptoms related to a severe aortic gradient, it may require prompt action. Typically patients with aortic stenosis are limited by shortness of breath at exertion. Because adaptation of lifestyle is common, it is crucial to recognize dyspnea due to aortic stenosis. Sometimes, a dramatic episode like syncope or cardiac arrhythmia occurs. Cardiac auscultation using a stethoscope is common in everyday practice throughout the health-care system, and the presence of a cardiac murmur may suggest an aortic stenosis. The same holds true for echocardiography (ECG), and signs of left ventricular hypertrophy may lead to further investigations.

2. Diagnostic tools

2.1 Echocardiography

Echocardiography is the cornerstone in identification and follow-up of aortic stenosis. It visualizes the calcification of the aortic valve, and the Doppler technique quantifies the left ventricular outflow gradient [1]. The aortic valve area can be estimated by calculation or planimetry but must be considered in conjunction with the mean gradient, wall thickness, ejection fraction, ventricular dimension, valve calcification, and hemodynamic parameters at the time of exam.

Four classes of aortic stenosis can be described:

- High-gradient aortic stenosis. Here the valve area is $<1\ cm^2$, and the mean gradient is >40 mmHg. This is clearly a severe aortic stenosis regardless of ejection fraction.

- Low-flow, low-gradient aortic stenosis with reduced ejection fraction. Dobutamine echocardiography may be useful in these situations; an aortic valve area above $1\ cm^2$ with flow normalization is suggestive of pseudosevere state.

IntechOpen

- Low-flow, low-gradient aortic stenosis with normal ejection fraction should be further evaluated if the area is <1 cm^2, especially in the elderly with ventricular hypertrophy and diminished left chamber size. Other imaging tools using computerized tomography are beneficial to assess calcification score [2, 3].

- Normal-flow, low-gradient aortic stenosis with normal ejection fraction and mean gradient <40 mmHg even though the valve area is <1 cm^2 is judged to be mild or moderate but not severe.

2.2 Exercise test

Evaluation of symptoms is related to the aortic stenosis that can be refined at an exercise test, typically ergometer bicycle test [4]. Using echocardiography at pharmacologically induced stress may reveal an increase in the pressure gradients [5]. Furthermore the response of ventricular function at exercise may give valuable information.

2.3 Miscellaneous imaging techniques

Multislice computerized tomography is nowadays an established method for quantification of valve calcification which is important in patients with low gradients. Furthermore computerized tomography offers excellent visualization of the aorta beyond the first part, the root. This is crucial in determination of preoperative anatomical assessment.

2.4 Laboratory markers

NT-proBNP is useful in follow-up of patients with aortic stenosis and is a complementary tool between intervals of echocardiography [6, 7].

3. Follow-up

Patients with aortic stenosis who are asymptomatic should undergo reevaluation every 6 months and should be asked to inform their physician the case of onset of symptoms. In mild to moderate aortic stenosis, evaluation every 3 years is reasonable but more often if significant calcification is assessed.

4. Treatment

4.1 Aortic stenosis without symptoms

While symptomatic severe aortic stenosis should be recommended intervention as rule of thumb, patients without symptoms are controversial. Still, the presence of an unequivocal severe aortic stenosis has not been proven to benefit from early intervention [8, 9]. Patients with reduced ejection fraction deemed to be secondary to aortic stenosis should not be refrained from an intervention. It is also reasonable to recommend intervention in cases of exercise-induced symptoms attributed to stenosis [10]. In the careful evaluation of asymptomatic patients, the following factors can be taken into account: massive hypertrophy, abnormal longitudinal left ventricular function, and pulmonary hypertension.

4.2 Pharmacological approach

Pharmacological therapy, including statins, has no impact on the disease progression in aortic stenosis. Nevertheless, concomitant hypertension should be treated. Patients who deteriorate into reduced ejection fraction should be subject to current heart failure optimization including beta-blocker, angiotensin-converting enzyme blocker/angiotensin receptor blocker, aldosterone receptor blocker, and rate/rhythm control if atrial fibrillation occurs.

4.3 Interventional approach

A patient with symptoms due to severe aortic stenosis should be evaluated for an interventional treatment. This is the only approach that will improve survival and relieve symptoms. In patients with an overall life expectancy of <12 months based on irreversible comorbidities, a conservative management is advocated.

The interventional mode is either surgical aortic valve replacement (SAVR) or transcatheter aortic valve implantation (TAVI). Based on the European Society Guidelines, a STS/EuroSCORE ≥4% favors TAVI and patients younger than 75 years based on limited long-term follow-up data of TAVI. In elderly patients, severe comorbidities (pulmonary or renal), considerable frailty, and those with restricted mobility, TAVI is preferred. In patients who previously underwent open-chest heart surgery, TAVI is advantageous due to adherent tissue which may complicate a second sternotomy.

4.4 Anatomical aspects: TAVI vs. SAVR

There are several factors that may be taken into account when choosing between TAVI and SAVR. A possible arterial approach is almost a prerequisite for TAVI, even though alternative routes may be an option. TAVI is the preferred method in patients who have sequele after chest radiation, porcelain aorta, risk of damage to grafting anastomosis following bypass surgery, and chest deformation. On the contrary, aortic root malfunction, thrombi in the aorta, and valve prosthesis mismatch are factors likely to favor TAVI.

SAVR should be performed in the case of concomitant need of other valve surgeries, aneurysm of the aorta, and septal hypertrophy requiring myectomy in hypertrophic cardiomyopathy.

4.5 Cardiac and extra-cardiac aspects: TAVI vs. SAVR

The individual risk should be assessed after careful evaluation and discussed between team members. The local resources and experience are important to be taken into account. In patients with high risk, TAVI is superior [11, 12]. Recently additional evidence points in the direction to favor TAVI in the majority of cases even in patients with low risk [13]. Notably, significant vascular complications, need of pacemaker implantation, and paravalvular regurgitation are more frequent for TAVI [14, 15]. SAVR is associated with more severe bleeding, acute renal failure, and atrial fibrillation. The risk of ischemic stroke seems to be similar [14, 15].

5. Future perspectives

The technical advancement of TAVI is expected to improve, and the increased volume is likely beneficial. However, long-term results over the decades are still lacking. Complications, including the need of pacemaker implant, require attention and further innovation of techniques besides increased experience. Nevertheless, careful clinical judgment in the individual case is always warranted.

Author details

Peter Magnusson[1,2]

1 Cardiology Research Unit, Department of Medicine, Karolinska Institute, Sweden

2 Centre for Research and Development, Uppsala University, Gävleborg, Gävle, Sweden

*Address all correspondence to: peter.magnusson@regiongavleborg.se

References

[1] Baumgartner H, Hung J, Bermejo J, Chambers JB, Edvardsen T, Goldstein S, et al. Focus update on the echocardiographic assessment of aortic valve stenosis: EAE/ASE recommendations for clinical practice. European Heart Journal Cardiovascular Imaging. 2017;**18**:254-275

[2] Cueff C, Serfaty JM, Cimadevilla C, Laissy JP, Himbert D, Tubach F, et al. Measurement of aortic valve calcification using multislice computed tomography: Correlation with haemodynamic severity of aortic stenosis and clinical implication for patients with low ejection fraction. Heart. 2011;**97**:721-726

[3] Clavel MA, Messika-Zeitoun D, Pibarot P, Aggarwal SR, Malouf J, Araoz PA, et al. The complex nature of discordant severe calcified aortic valve disease grading: New insights from combined Doppler echocardiographic and computed tomographic study. Journal of the American College of Cardiology. 2013;**62**:2329-2338

[4] Rafique AM, Biner S, Ray I, Forrester JS, Tolstrup K, Siegel RJ. Meta-analysis of prognostic value of stress testing in patients with asymptomatic severe aortic stenosis. The American Journal of Cardiology. 2009;**104**:972-977

[5] Marechaux S, Hachicha Z, Bellouin A, Dumesnil JG, Meimoun P, Pasquet A, et al. Usefulness of exercise-stress echocardiography for risk stratification of true asymptomatic patients with aortic valve stenosis. European Heart Journal. 2010;**31**:1390-1397

[6] Bergler-Klein J, Klaar U, Heger M, Rosenhek R, Mundigler G, Gabriel H, et al. Natriuretic peptides predict symptom-free survival and postoperative outcome in severe aortic stenosis. Circulation. 2004;**109**:2302-2308

[7] Clavel MA, Malouf J, Michelena HI, Suri RM, Jaffe AS, Mahoney DW, et al. B-type natriuretic peptide clinical activation in aortic stenosis: Impact on long-term survival. Journal of the American College of Cardiology. 2014;**63**:2016-2025

[8] Rosenhek R, Binder T, Porenta G, Lang I, Christ G, Schemper M, et al. Predictors of outcome in severe, asymptomatic aortic stenosis. The New England Journal of Medicine. 2000;**343**:611-617

[9] Genereux P, Stone GW, O'Gara PT, Marquis-Gravel G, Redfors B, Giustino G, et al. Natural history, diagnostic approaches, and therapeutic strategies for patients with asymptomatic severe aortic stenosis. Journal of the American College of Cardiology. 2016;**67**:2263-2288

[10] Das P, Rimington H, Chambers J. Exercise testing to stratify risk in aortic stenosis. European Heart Journal. 2005;**26**:1309-1313

[11] Leon MB, Smith CR, Mack M, Miller DC, Moses JW, Svensson LG, et al. PARTNER trial investigators. Transcatheter aortic-valve implantation for aortic stenosis in patients who cannot undergo surgery. The New England Journal of Medicine. 2010;**363**:1597-1607

[12] Deeb GM, Reardon MJ, Chetcuti S, Patel HJ, Grossman PM, Yakubov SJ, et al. CoreValve US clinical investigators. 3-year outcomes in high-risk patients who underwent surgical or transcatheter aortic valve replacement. Journal of the American College of Cardiology. 2016;**67**:2565-2574

[13] Popma JJ, Deeb GM, Yakubov SJ, Mumtaz M, Gada H, O'Hair D, et al. Transcatheter aortic-valve replacement with a self-expanding valve in low-risk

patients. The New England Journal of Medicine. 2019;**380**:1706-1715

[14] Siontis GC, Praz F, Pilgrim T, Mavridis D, Verma S, Salanti G, et al. Transcatheter aortic valve implantation vs. surgical aortic valve replacement for treatment of severe aortic stenosis: A meta-analysis of randomized trials. European Heart Journal. 2016;**37**:3503-3512

[15] Reardon MJ, Van Mieghem NM, Popma JJ, Kleiman NS, Sondergaard L, Mumtaz M, et al. SURTAVI Investigators. Surgical or transcatheter aortic-valve replacement in intermediate-risk patients. The New England Journal of Medicine. 2017;**376**:1321-1331

Chapter 2

Low Flow Low Gradient Severe Aortic Stenosis: Diagnosis and Treatment

Faeez Mohamad Ali, Vindhya Wilson and Rajesh Nair

Abstract

Approximately 40% of patients with aortic stenosis (AS) show discordant Doppler-echocardiographic parameters with aortic valve area (AVA) <1 cm^2 and/or index iAVA <0.6 cm^2/m^2 (consistent with severe AS) and the mean gradient (MG) <40 mmHg, consistent with mild/moderate AS. Accurate diagnosis of true severe low flow low gradient AS versus pseudo-severe aortic stenosis is important for prognosis and optimal timing for intervention. Doppler echocardiography using intravenous low dose dobutamine challenge is widely used for differentiating pseudo-severe from true severe aortic stenosis. However, relying on echocardiography alone may have limitations in accurate diagnosis. Reliable diagnosis using echocardiography is dependent on multiple factors like the angle of interrogation of the aortic jet, the assumption that the LVOT area is circular in cross section, optimal echo windows, the presence of underlying subclinical coronary artery disease prior to dobutamine challenge etc. In this chapter, we describe non-invasive and invasive strategies to assess the aortic valve using dobutamine stress. Direct measurement of gradients across the aortic valve while estimating the change in cardiac output and aortic valve area with increments of dobutamine infusion dose is complementary, safe and useful when conventional echocardiography techniques are inconclusive. Finally, the chapter describes effective strategies of treatment for low gradient severe aortic stenosis, including the role for diagnostic balloon valvuloplasty, in the era of transcatheter valve replacement (TAVR).

Keywords: balloon aortic valvuloplasty, dobutamine stress test, low flow low gradient severe aortic stenosis, pseudo-severe aortic stenosis, trans-catheter aortic valve replacement

1. Introduction

Degenerative calcific aortic stenosis (AS) is the commonest primary valvular heart disease responsible for approximately 85,000 valve replacement procedures and 15,000 deaths per year in North America [1].

The diagnosis and staging of AS is primarily based on symptoms and Doppler echocardiography. AS is considered severe when the patient has a mean transvalvular gradient >40 mmHg, a peak aortic jet velocity >4 m/s, an aortic valve area (AVA) <1.0 cm^2, indexed aortic valve area (iAVA) <0.6 cm^2/m^2 and a dimensionless velocity index <0.25 [2–4].

However, in up to 40% of patients with AS, there is discordance between aortic valve area (<1 cm^2 suggesting severe AS) and transvalvular gradients (<40 mmHg suggesting non-severe AS) on Doppler echocardiography [5–7]. These patients are referred to as having "low gradient" severe AS. Most of these patients have a "low flow state" across the aortic valve, which is defined as an indexed stroke volume <35 ml/m^2. Many of these patients may be quite advanced in the natural history of severe AS. Despite challenges in establishing accurate diagnosis, "low gradient" severe AS patients tend to have poorer outcomes compared to patients with "high gradient" severe AS. This chapter describes the etiology, classification, diagnosis and management options of low flow low gradient (LFLG) severe AS.

2. Classification of aortic stenosis

All major guidelines have classified aortic stenosis based on hemodynamic parameters, symptoms and the left ventricular (LV) systolic function (**Figure 1**). According to the American College of Cardiology/American Heart Association, severe aortic stenosis is classified into asymptomatic severe AS (stage C) and symptomatic severe AS (stage D). Asymptomatic severe AS depending on LV function is further sub classified into stage C1—with normal LV function and stage C2—with reduced LV function (left ventricular ejection fraction (LVEF) <50%). Symptomatic severe AS is sub classified into three stages depending on blood flow across the aortic valve and hemodynamic characteristics (**Figure 2**). Normal flow (>35 ml/m^2), high gradient (>40 mmHg), severe AS (AVA <1 cm^2/iAVA <0.6 cm/m^2) is the most easily recognized entity with little diagnostic confusion (stage D1).

Low flow low gradient (LFLG) severe aortic stenosis (stages D2 and D3) represents an advanced stage in the hemodynamic spectrum of severe AS with poor prognosis and higher surgical morbidity and mortality than normal flow high gradient severe AS [8–12].

Although not incorporated into guidelines some authors recognize another variant called normal flow low gradient severe AS. This is a relatively poorly defined entity with unclear pathophysiology. Apart from measurement errors, one proposed explanation is that these patients have reduced arterial compliance (stiff arteries), which leads to a faster arterial wave reflection from the periphery. The

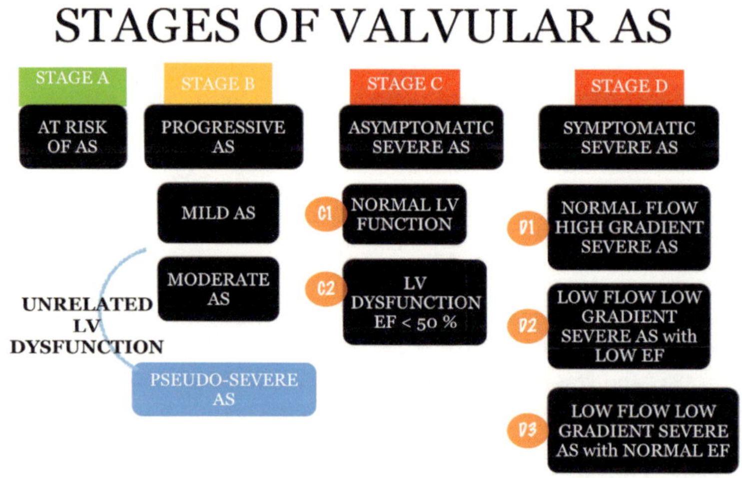

Figure 1.
Stage of aortic stenosis—adapted and modified from Nishimura et al. [2].

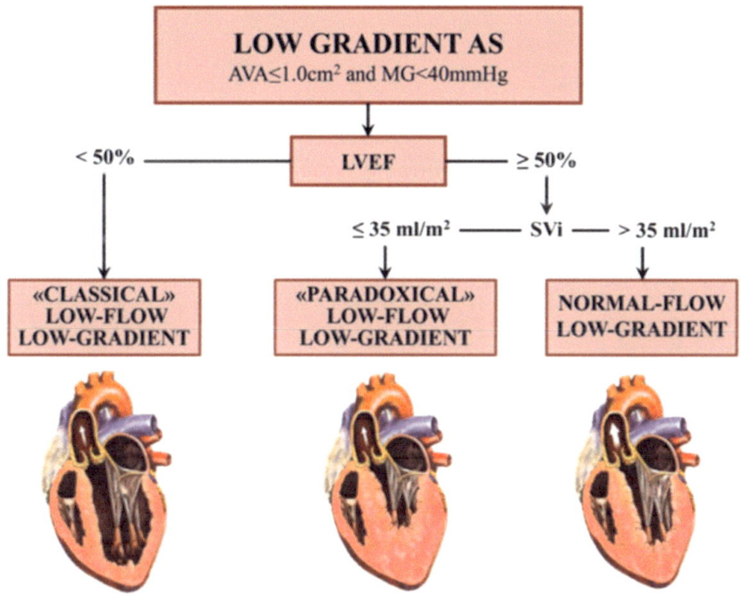

Figure 2.
Subtypes of low-gradient aortic stenosis. AS, aortic stenosis; AVA, aortic valve area; LVEF, left ventricular ejection fraction; MG, mean transvalvular gradient; SVi, stroke volume index. Reproduced with permission from Clavel et al. [32].

early reflection of the arterial wave at the end of systole may dampen the transvalvular gradients, independent of transvalvular flow. This phenomenon may, in part, explain the small AVA and low gradient discordance observed in patients with normal flow, low gradient severe AS.

2.1 Low flow low gradient severe AS with reduced ejection fraction (stage D2)

This entity is found in about 5–10% of patients with severe AS. It is more prevalent in men, and is very often associated with coronary artery disease [13]. LFLG severe AS is defined as indexed stroke volume <35 ml/m^2, LVEF <50%, AVA <1.0 cm^2/iAVA <0.6 cm^2/m^2 and mean aortic valve gradient <40 mmHg [2]. As severe AS progresses over several years, the left ventricle responds to the increase in afterload by concentric left ventricular hypertrophy. This compensatory mechanism helps the left ventricle pump against an increase in afterload as well as offset the increase in wall tension. The compensatory mechanism is reflected in the natural history of aortic stenosis where patients with severe AS who are truly asymptomatic have a relatively long symptom free period. However onset of symptoms indicates a significant turning point in the natural history with poor prognosis when left untreated (**Figure 3**). The average life expectancy for patients with severe AS is 2 years for those with shortness of breath, 3 years for patients with syncope, and 5 years for those with angina [16].

Patients who start out as normal flow high gradient severe AS eventually transform into LFLG severe AS with reduced LVEF through a number mechanisms (**Figure 4**). The long standing persistent left ventricular hypertrophy leads to oxygen supply demand mismatch, reduced capillary density, chronic subendocardial ischemia and interstitial fibrosis. Another important reason for LV dysfunction is coexistent coronary artery disease seen in a majority of these patients—49–76% [8, 9, 12].

Eventually the left ventricle fails to keep up with the high pressure gradients and decompensates due to the afterload mismatch. The LV dilates, stroke volumes drops

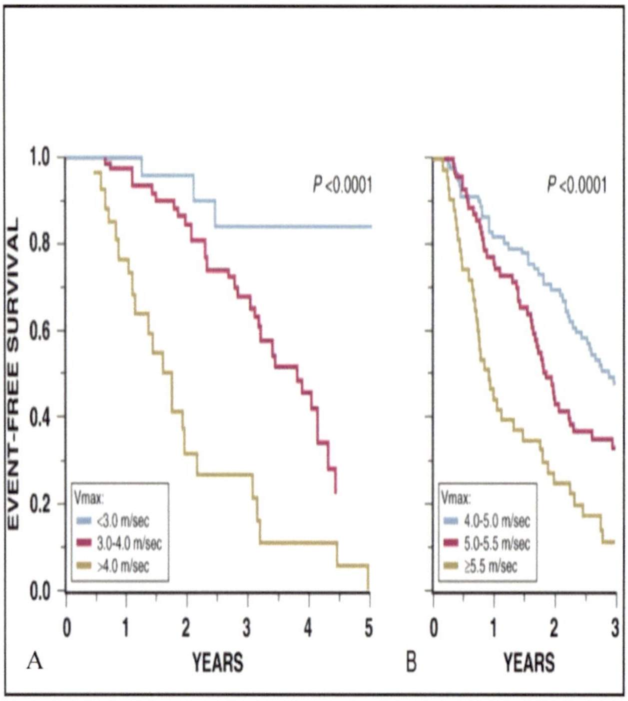

Figure 3.
(A) Natural history as reflected by event-free survival in asymptomatic patients with AS. Initial aortic jet velocity (Vmax) stratifies patients according to the likelihood that symptoms requiring valve replacement will develop over time [14]. (B) Outcomes with very severe AS. Kaplan-Meier event-free survival rate for patients with a peak aortic jet velocity of 4.0 m/s or greater [15]. In both A and B, most "events" consisted of the onset of symptoms warranting aortic valve replacement.

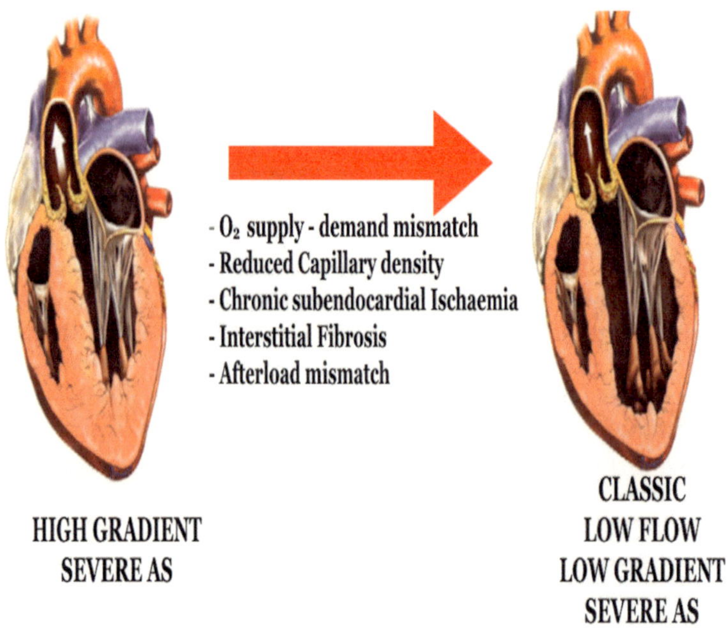

Figure 4.
Factors leading to transformation of high gradient severe aortic stenosis to low flow low gradient severe aortic stenosis with reduced ejection fraction.

and LVEF falls. As the flow across the stenosed aortic valve declines, the ability of the valve to open (which is flow dependent) reduces and hence the calculated aortic valve area is low. The pressure gradients across the valve are measured by modified Bernoulli's equation ($P = 4V^2$, P, transaortic valve pressure gradient; V, maximum velocity of the aortic jet). Since flow velocities decline along with the stroke volume, the measured pressure gradients also drop exponentially. This leads to LFLG severe AS, with overall poor prognosis and a consensus class IIa recommendation for aortic valve replacement (AVR).

2.2 Low flow low gradient severe AS with preserved left ventricular ejection fraction (stage D3)

As opposed to patients with "classic" LFLG AS with reduced LVEF, those with "paradoxical" LFLG AS have preserved LVEF. This entity is defined as an LVEF >50%, the presence of a low flow (stroke volume index <35 ml/m^2), an AVA <1.0 cm^2, an iAVA <0.6 cm^2/m^2, and a mean aortic valve gradient <40 mmHg [2, 5, 17]. LFLG pattern is seen in 5–15% of patients with severe AS and is more prevalent in women and elderly patients. These patients have excessive LV hypertrophy in response to the hemodynamic stress. As a result they have small LV cavities and hence a low stroke volumes despite the preserved LVEF. Other factors (**Figure 5**) that contribute to low forward flow across the aortic valve include mitral regurgitation/stenosis, tricuspid regurgitation/stenosis, atrial fibrillation and infiltrative cardiomyopathies like amyloidosis. Paradoxical LFLG AS shares clinical, pathological and hemodynamic similarities with heart failure with preserved ejection fraction. Both conditions are characterized by significant concentric left ventricular hypertrophy

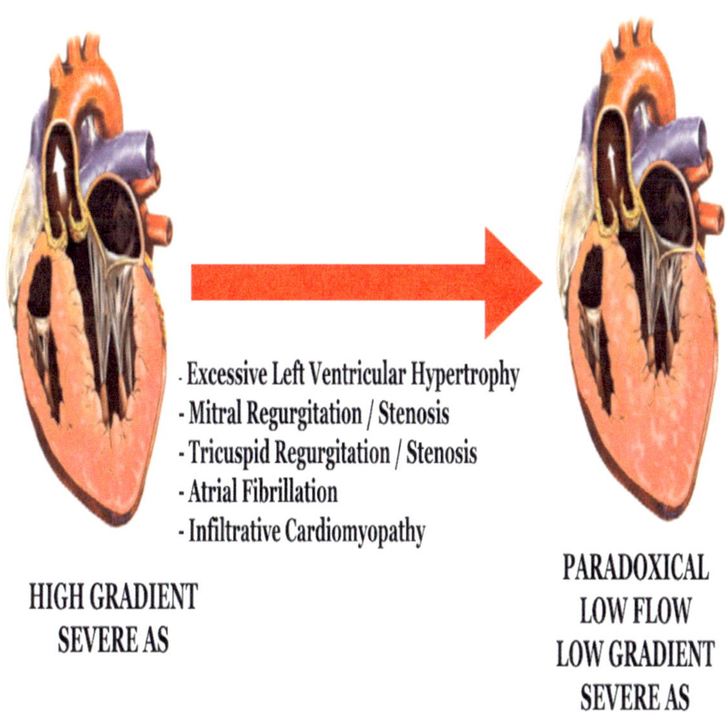

Figure 5.
Factors leading to transformation of high gradient severe aortic stenosis to paradoxical low flow low gradient severe aortic stenosis.

leading to small cavity size and restrictive physiology. In addition there is marked reduction in intrinsic LV systolic function that may not be apparent by routinely used echocardiographic indices. Global longitudinal strain is a more sensitive parameter that helps unmask the apparently normal LVEF in these patients. It is reduced to a larger extent due to fibrosis along the subendocardial layer. These findings suggest that paradoxical LFLG AS is a more advanced stage in the hemodynamic spectrum of severe AS [5, 18, 19] and classified in guidelines as stage D3.

2.3 Moderate aortic stenosis with left ventricular dysfunction—"pseudo-severe" aortic stenosis

One of the main challenges in the diagnosis of LFLG severe AS is distinguishing it from pseudo-severe AS, i.e., moderate AS with underlying LV dysfunction, unrelated to aortic stenosis. In this case, the primary culprit is LV dysfunction; typically due to associated cardiomyopathy (ischemic or idiopathic) or myocarditis. The myopathic ventricle fails to generate adequate blood flow to open the aortic valve sufficiently, hence overestimating severity of AS on echocardiography. At the same time, the gradients across the aortic valve are low related to lower transvalvular flow. This produces a hemodynamic picture similar to LFLG severe AS. Studies have shown that in patients with pseudo-severe AS, the 5-year survival with medical therapy is better than in true severe AS and comparable with that of propensity matched patients with heart failure with reduced ejection fraction and no evidence of valve disease (**Figure 6**) [20].

Paradoxically, moderate aortic stenosis for a normal ventricle may be functionally more significant for the myopathic ventricle. Some studies have suggested that moderate AS may have a detrimental effect on outcomes in patients with coexistent LV dysfunction. This concept raises the hypothesis that aortic valve replacement (AVR) may be beneficial in such patients [21, 22]. Trans-catheter Aortic Valve

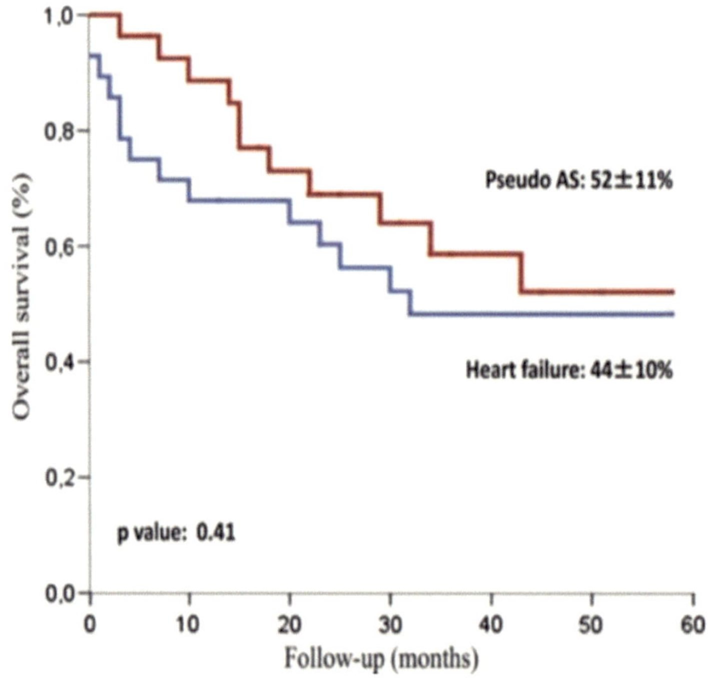

Figure 6.
Kaplan-Meier survival estimates under conservative treatment among 28 patients with pseudo-severe aortic stenosis and 28 propensity-matched patients with systolic heart failure. Reproduced with permission from Fougères et al. [20].

Replacement to UNload the Left ventricle in patients with ADvanced heart failure (TAVR UNLOAD) trial is designed to test the above hypothesis. Patients with heart failure with reduced ejection fraction and moderate AS confirmed by resting and/or dobutamine stress echocardiography are randomized to optimized heart failure therapy alone versus optimized heart failure therapy plus transcatheter AVR.

3. Diagnosis of low flow low gradient severe aortic stenosis

Transthoracic echocardiogram is the gold standard to detect the "low flow state" across the aortic valve. Accurate Doppler echocardiographic measurements of stroke volume, AVA, and gradient are important to minimize underestimation of severe AS or an overestimation of moderate AS.

3.1 Echocardiographic caveats in estimating AS severity

Typically Doppler echocardiographic assessment is operator dependent. Optimal alignment of the continuous wave Doppler beam with the direction of the aortic flow jet is crucial to accurately quantify aortic valve gradient, aortic valve area and thereby severity of AS. The apical window detects peak velocity in 40% of cases where as the right parasternal window picks up peak velocity in 50% of cases [23]. A multiwindow approach is recommended which includes apical, right parasternal, suprasternal and right supraclavicular windows.

The most common technical pitfall that may lead to an erroneous diagnosis of low-flow state and overestimation of AS severity is underestimation of the left ventricular outflow tract (LVOT) diameter. The effective AVA is determined by the continuity equation method (**Figure** 7), which is based on the principle that the flow across the left ventricular outflow tract should be equal to the flow across the aortic valve. Since the LVOT diameter is squared in the equation, an underestimation of the LVOT diameter may lead to underestimation of valve area and thus the false conclusion that the patient has LFLG severe AS when, in fact, the patient has normal flow and/or moderate AS.

The 2009 European Association of Echocardiography/American Society of Echocardiography guidelines suggest measuring the diameter and velocity 5–10 mm below the aortic annulus. However, recent studies suggest measuring the LVOT diameter inner-edge-to-inner-edge from the base of the right coronary cusp anteriorly to the commissure posteriorly [24, 25]. From a practical standpoint, an easy way to measure the LVOT diameter is to assess the pulse wave Doppler signal from the distal to proximal LVOT in the apical view. The LVOT velocity time integral is then measured just below the point where aliasing is seen, when the flow signals are smooth with sharp borders. The LVOT diameter is ideally measured at this point in the parasternal long axis view (**Figure 8**).

3.1.1 Dobutamine stress echocardiography

Once technical errors in measurement are ruled out, it is essential to distinguish LFLG true severe AS from pseudo-severe AS. deFilippi et al. [26] were the first to demonstrate that low dose (up to 20 μg/kg/min) dobutamine stress echocardiography (DSE) may be used in these patients to distinguish true versus pseudo-severe stenosis. The use of DSE for this purpose has received a class IIa (level of evidence: B) recommendation in the American College of Cardiology/American Heart Association-European Society of Cardiology (ACC/AHA-ESC/EACTS) guidelines [1–3], and a similar protocol has also been used for invasive assessment in cardiac catheterization laboratory by Nishimura et al. [27].

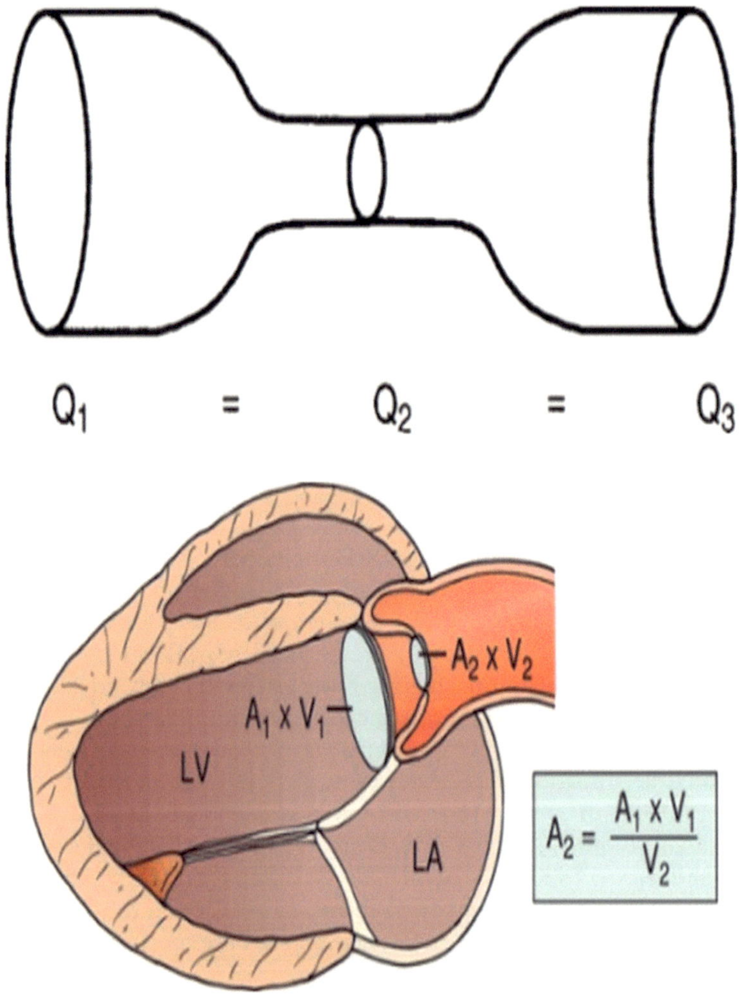

Figure 7.
Continuity equation, formula to calculate aortic valve area. The LVOT is assumed to be cross sectional in area.

Dobutamine recruits myocardial contractility in normal and hibernating myocardium, thus enhancing stroke volume and transvalvular flow. This is referred to as "stroke volume reserve." Patients with more than 20% rise in stroke volume at peak dobutamine levels are referred to as having stroke volume reserve. When the flow across the valve increases, depending on the underlying condition, one of two possibilities occurs. If the patient has true severe AS, the valve being intrinsically restricted cannot open up further. In this case the transaortic gradients will increase with little or no change in aortic valve area. On the other hand in patients with pseudo-severe AS, aortic valve area increases significantly (>0.6 cm^2/m^2) with little or no change in trans-aortic gradients (**Figure 9**).

Though not incorporated into guidelines, in our experience, DSE can also be used in patients with LFLG severe AS with preserved LVEF. Dobutamine is able to recruit the subendocardial longitudinally oriented myocardial fibers and further increase transvalvular flow. Studies have estimated that about 30–40% of patients with LFLG severe AS may not have adequate stroke volume reserve (<20% rise in stroke volume with peak dobutamine stress) [9, 21, 26–28]. They have higher operative mortality (22–33%) than those with flow reserve (5–8%) [9]. However the presence or absence of flow reserve cannot be used to predict recovery of LV function after valve replacement

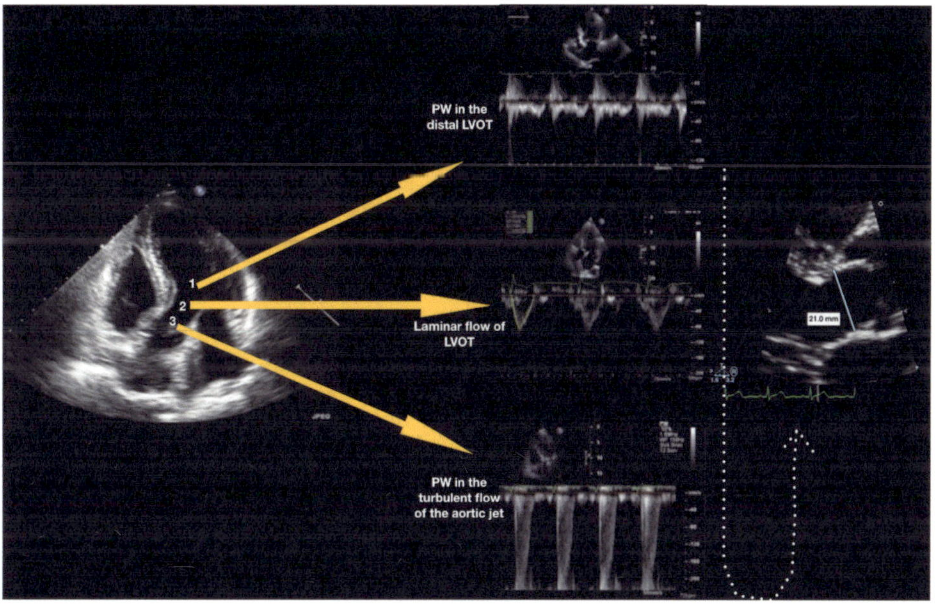

Figure 8.
The pulse wave Doppler is walked from the distal to proximal LVOT. At point 3, aliasing is noted suggesting that the Doppler signal is within the turbulent aortic jet. The pulse wave Doppler is moved just distal to point 3 (at point 2) where laminar LVOT velocities are seen. The LVOT VTI is measured at this point and the LVOT diameter at this corresponding point in the parasternal long axis view.

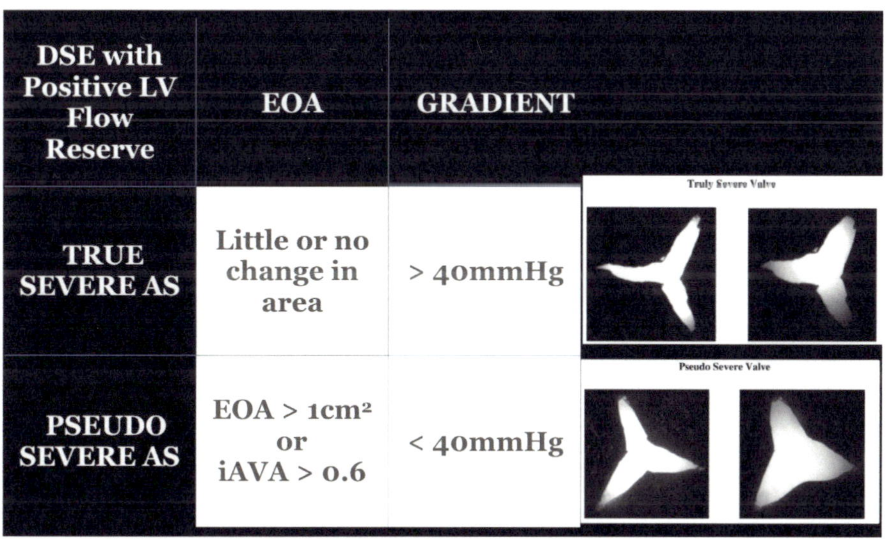

DSE with Positive LV Flow Reserve	EOA	GRADIENT	
TRUE SEVERE AS	Little or no change in area	> 40mmHg	Truly Severe Valve
PSEUDO SEVERE AS	EOA > 1cm² or iAVA > 0.6	< 40mmHg	Pseudo Severe Valve

Figure 9.
In the presence of stroke volume reserve, if the valve area remains more or less constant with increase in gradient >40 mmHg, it is suggestive of true severe AS. On the other hand, if the valve area increases with no significant change in gradients, it is suggestive of pseudo severe AS.

and cannot be used to determine long term prognosis. The French Multicenter Study of LFLG AS reported that, in patients with no LV flow reserve who survived surgical aortic valve replacement (SAVR) had similar improvement in post-operative LVEF and late survival rate compared to patients with preserved LV flow reserve [29] (**Figure 10**).

These findings suggest that DSE is useful to distinguish true severe from pseudo-severe AS and estimate operative risk. However, DES does not predict recovery of

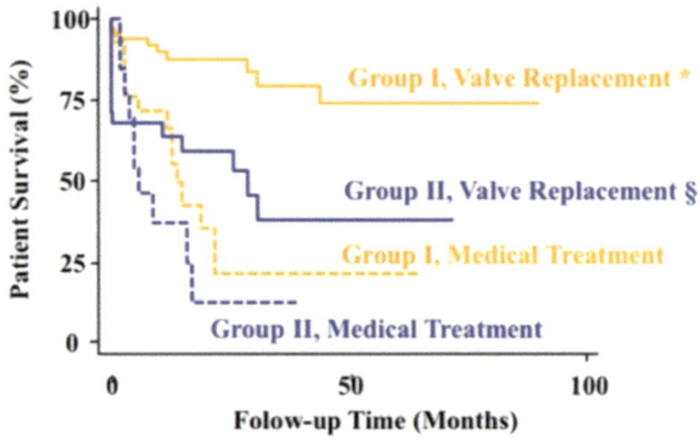

Figure 10.
*Patients with no LV flow (contractile) reserve (Group II) defined as 20% increase in stroke volume during DSE have markedly reduced survival compared with those with LV flow reserve (Group I), regardless of the type of treatment. Aortic valve replacement is associated with dramatic improvement in survival in patients with LV flow reserve and a trend for better survival in those with no flow reserve. *p 0.001 versus medical; §p 0.07 versus medical. Adapted with permission from Monin et al. [9].*

LV function, improvement in symptom status, and late survival after SAVR [9, 13, 30]. Though the absence of flow reserve portends higher perioperative mortality, DSE should only be used as a diagnostic modality. The absence of LV flow reserve should not exclude patients for AVR [9, 12].

3.1.2 Projected effective orifice area

DSE results maybe inconclusive in 30–40% due to inadequate stroke volume reserve [9, 13]. In this patient subset, the investigators of the TOPAS (Truly or Pseudo-Severe Aortic Stenosis) study proposed to calculate the projected effective orifice area (EOA) that would have occurred at a standardized flow rate of 250 ml/s (EOAProj) [21, 31] (**Figure 11**). This parameter, standardized for flow, has been shown to better predict the actual hemodynamic severity of the valve stenosis and the clinical outcome of patients with classical or paradoxical LFLG AS, as compared with standard stress echocardiography parameters [8, 21, 33]. A projected AVA <1.0 cm^2 confirms the presence of true severe AS (**Figure 11**). Some patients may not have an adequate increase in stroke volume but nevertheless will have an increase in transvalvular flow rate due to shortening of ejection time. The phase III of the TOPAS study is currently underway and is expected to be completed by 2022.

3.1.3 CT calcium score of the aortic valve

About 15–20% of patients may have inconclusive results from DSE and may not have adequate transvalvular flow rate to calculate projected effective orifice area. DSE can be used in patients with paradoxical LFLG AS; however, some patients with very small LV cavities can develop dynamic LVOT obstruction and hypotension. For such patients, an alternative method to assess aortic stenosis severity is proposed.

Multi detector computerized tomography (MDCT) scan without contrast can accurately quantify calcium distribution along the AV leaflets. Calcium burden along the AV leaflets has been shown to correlate with severity of aortic stenosis [34]. It is an anatomical test independent of hemodynamics, blood flow and does not require administration of contrast or any stress agents. For the quantitation of calcification, a non-contrast MDCT scan during trained end-inspiration breath-hold is performed. Radiation exposure for such an examination is <3 mSV. The amount of calcification in the region of the aortic valve is quantitated using the

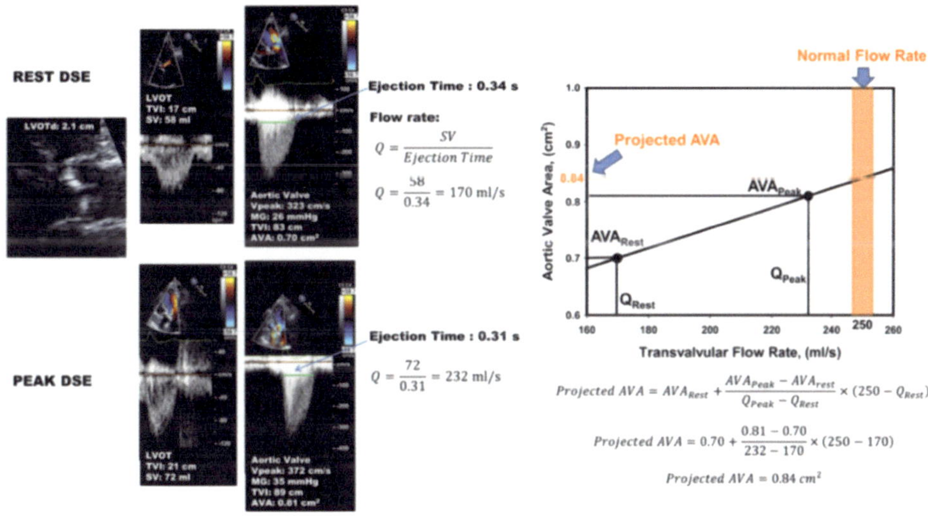

Figure 11.
DSE in a patient with low flow low gradient state across the aortic valve. Even with dobutamine the valve area is 0.81 cm² and the mean gradient is still <40 mmHg. Due to inconclusive results, the projected effective orifice area is calculated at a normalized flow rate of 250 ml/s which is 0.84 cm² suggesting the presence of true severe AS. Adapted with permission from Clavel et al. [32].

modified Agatston method, in which calcification is defined as four adjacent pixels with a density >130 Hounsfield Units [35]. The aortic valve calcium score measured by MDCT strongly correlates with hemodynamic severity, the progression rate, and the clinical outcomes of AS patients [34, 36, 37]. Women tend to develop less calcification for the same degree of severity of stenosis. Cut off values for valve calcification to differentiate severe versus non-severe AS in men is >2000 AU and in women >1200 AU [34, 38]. The same approach should be applied when using cutoff point for aortic valve calcium density (i.e., calcium score indexed to LVOT area): >500 AU/cm^2 in men versus >300 AU/cm^2 in women [34–38] (**Figure 12**).

It is important to note that MDCT grossly underestimates valve fibrosis and hence significantly underestimates severe AS in younger patients [39]. Hence this technique may be used in older patients where the degenerative aortic valve pathology is driven by valve calcification.

3.1.4 Invasive assessment of aortic stenosis in the catheterization laboratory

3.1.4.1 Pitfalls of echocardiography in diagnosis of AS

The advent of echocardiography revolutionized the field of cardiology providing hemodynamic data that could only be previously obtained by invasive cardiac catheterization. However echocardiographic derivations are based on some basic assumptions, which might not be reliable for all patient anatomy. Furthermore, there are limitations on subjective assessment by personnel with varying experience. Doppler measurements are dependent on the angle of insinuation of the sound waves against the jet of blood flow across the aortic valve (**Figure 13**). Depending on the restriction along the leaflet coaptation edges, the jet of blood through the stenosed AV, can be eccentric. This makes it almost impossible to align the continuous wave Doppler perpendicular to the jet. The peak velocity is inversely proportional to the cosine of the angle of insinuation. Even a 1° off axis tilt may reduce the peak velocity by 0.04 m/s representing an error of 1%, considering a cut off value of 4 m/s for severe aortic stenosis. When the estimated velocity is squared to calculate pressure gradient across the aortic valve, any error is exponentially increased.

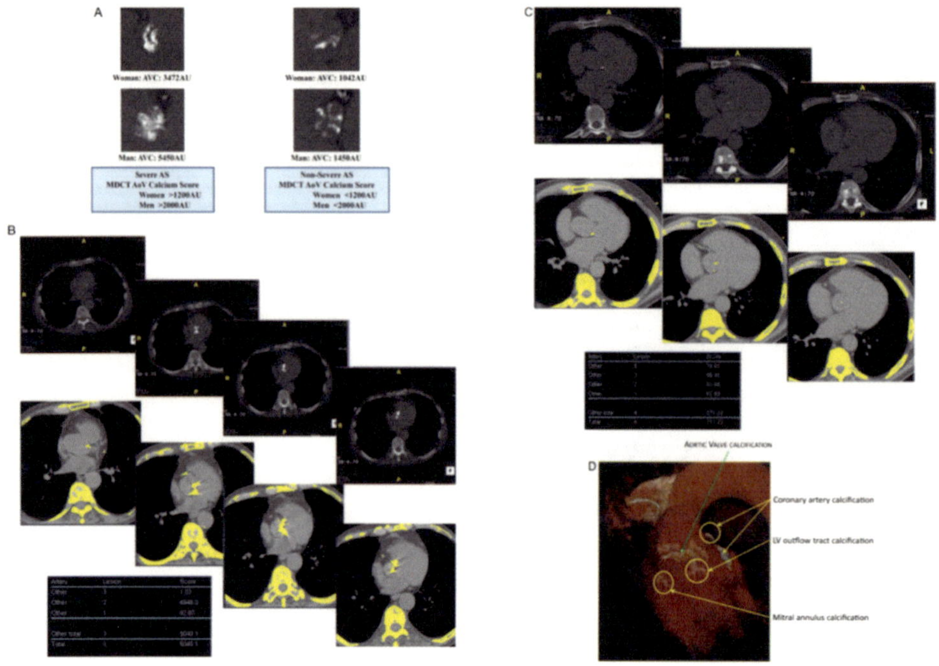

Figure 12.
Quantitation of aortic valve calcium by multi-detector computed tomography for the assessment of stenosis severity in low-gradient aortic stenosis. (A) Multi-detector computed tomography can be used to quantitate aortic valve calcification by the modified Agatston method. With this method, calcification is defined as four adjacent pixels with density 0.130 Hounsfield units. Different cut-point values of valve calcium score should be used in women (0.1200 AU) versus men (0.2000 AU) to differentiate true-severe versus pseudo-severe stenosis in low-flow, low-gradient aortic stenosis. (B) Serial multi-detector computed tomography slices at the level of the aortic valve showing a severely calcified valve with a calcium score of 5040 AU consistent with true-severe aortic stenosis. Calcified areas are displayed in yellow in the bottom images. (C) Mild calcification (score 271 AU) consistent with pseudo-severe aortic stenosis. (D) Pitfalls in the assessment of aortic valve calcification by multi-detector computed tomography. For the calculation of calcium score, it is important to only include aortic valve calcification and exclude calcification of aorta, coronary arteries, LVOT, and mitral annulus. Adapted with permission from Clavel et al. [32].

Another common limitation of echocardiography is the assumption that LVOT is circular in cross section, when in fact it is circular in only 1–2% of cases (**Figure 14**). The LVOT is a three-dimensional (3D) dynamic structure that is often elliptical, with the antero-posterior dimension representing the smaller minor axis diameter, as compared with the generally larger diameter in the sagittal plane. Hence, 2D echocardiography may underestimate the LVOT area compared with 3D imaging modalities such as 3D echocardiography, MDCT, or cardiac magnetic resonance [40–43]. To overcome the potential underestimation of the LVOT diameter and stroke volume and AVA by 2D echocardiography, the use of a hybrid approach has been suggested, where the LVOT area is measured by MDCT or 3D echocardiography and the LVOT and aortic flow velocities are measured by Doppler echocardiography [43, 44]. However, it is also important to note, the AVA value generally used to define severe AS <1.0 cm^2, has been established and validated by outcome studies, where AVA was measured by standard 2D Doppler-echocardiography [2, 4]. A recent study demonstrated that the hybrid approach systematically overestimates the LVOT area and thus AVA. The best discriminative hybrid AVA to predict mortality in patients with AS under medical treatment was larger (1.2 cm^2) versus the Doppler-echocardiographic AVA (1.0 cm^2) [43].

Finally, it becomes difficult to obtain LVOT velocity time integral when there is associated subaortic fixed or dynamic obstruction contributing to transvalvular gradients.

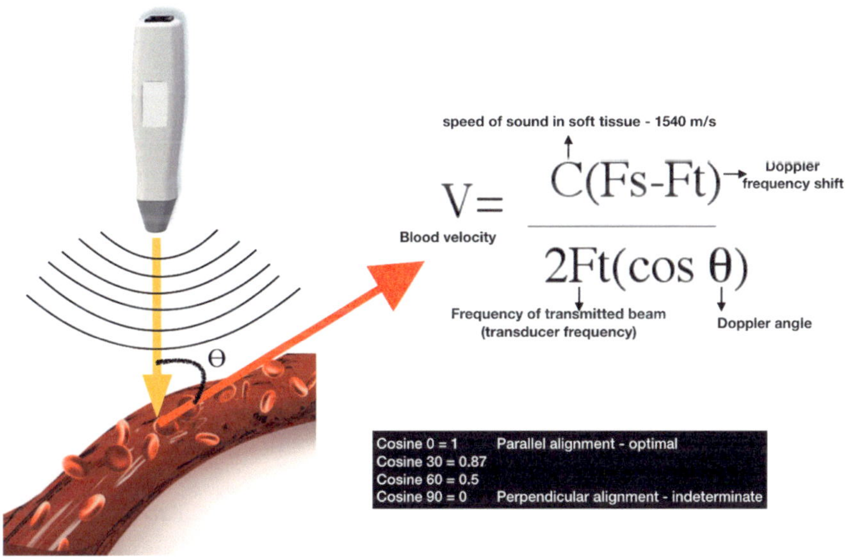

Figure 13.
Doppler measurements are angle dependent. For optimal values the angle of insinuation should be parallel/antiparallel (0 or 180°) to the flow of blood. As the Doppler angle increases, the measured velocities decrease, thus underestimating velocities.

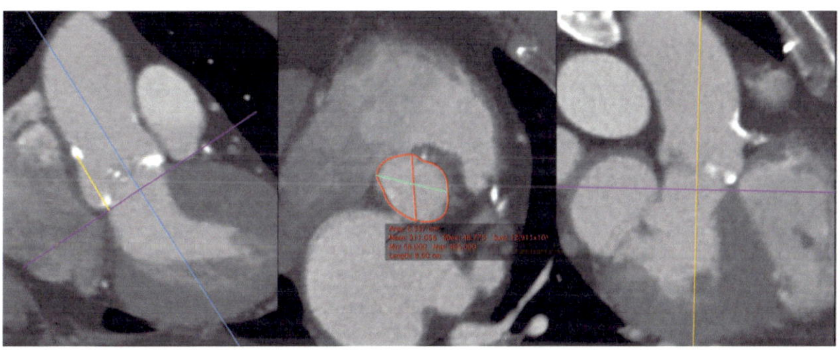

Figure 14.
CT showing elliptical shape of the LVOT.

3.1.4.2 Invasive assessment of severe AS

Currently invasive measurement is recommended only when non-invasive tests are inconclusive, the patient has poor echo windows or when there is significant discrepancy between the patient's clinical symptoms and echocardiographic data. **Figure 15** shows the steps of invasive assessment of aortic stenosis in the catheterization lab. Ideally simultaneous pressure gradients are measured by obtaining dual arterial access. Single arterial puncture may also be used for diagnosis by inserting a 7F long sheath reaching the ascending aorta from where pressure can be transduced from the side port of the long sheath. The pressure from the left ventricle should be transduced through a 5F pigtail catheter inserted into the left ventricle through the long sheath. The cardiac output is measured either by thermodilution using a Swan Ganz catheter or by Fick's principle. Dobutamine stress can be achieved using incremental doses, infused through a venous sheath. Cardiac output, mean gradient across the aortic valve, aortic valve area and iAVA is calculated after at least 2 minutes of incremental dobutamine infusion [27].

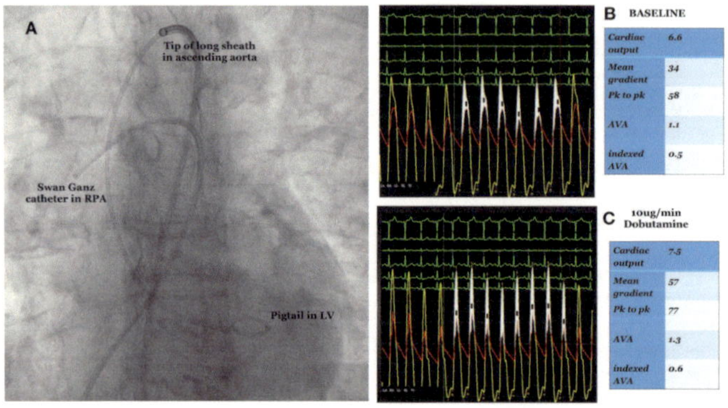

Figure 15.
Invasive assessment of low flow gradient AS in the Cathlab. Panel A shows the initial setup of the catheters. A 7F long sheath is positioned with its tip in the ascending aorta from where aortic pressures are transduced. A 5F pigtail is positioned in the LV through the long sheath to measure LV pressures. A Swan Ganz catheter is positioned in the pulmonary artery to measure cardiac output at each stage. Panel B—at baseline the patient is shown to have an indexed valve area of 0.5 cm², with a mean gradient of 34 mmHg across the aortic valve. Panel C—with 10 μg/min of dobutamine, the trans-aortic gradients increase from 34 to 57 mmHg with no significant change in indexed valve area suggesting the presence of true severe AS.

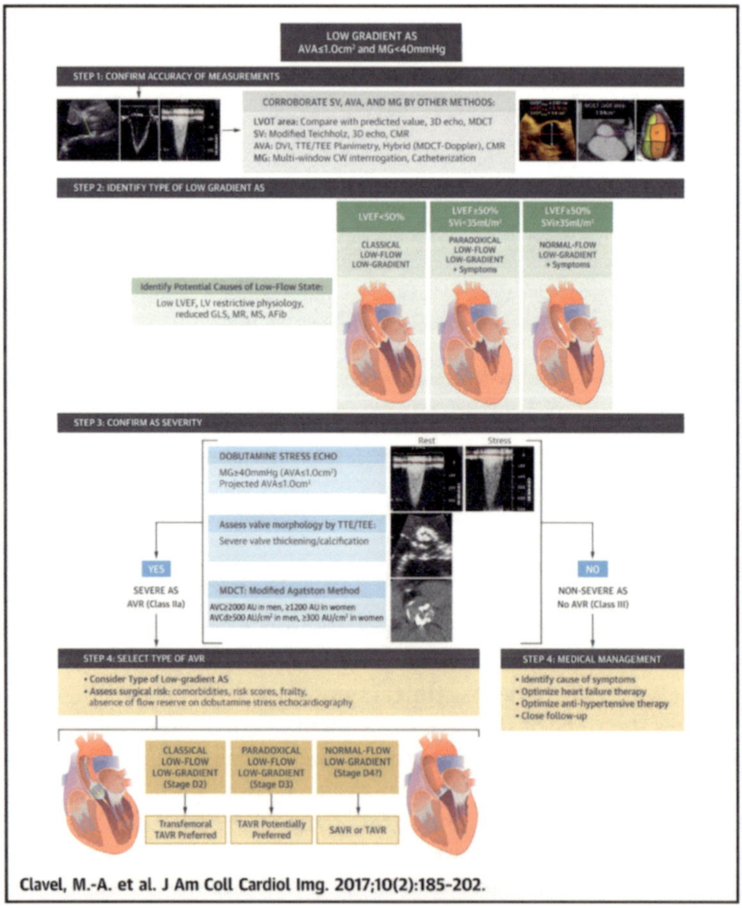

Figure 16.
Four-step algorithm for the diagnostic and therapeutic management of low-gradient AS. AVC ¼ aortic valve calcification; AVCd ¼ aortic valve calcification density; AVR ¼ aortic valve replacement; CMR ¼ cardiac magnetic resonance; MDCT ¼ multi-detector computed tomography; RCT ¼ randomized controlled trial; TEE ¼ transesophageal echocardiography; TTE ¼ transthoracic echocardiography. Reproduced with permission from Clavel et al. [1].

Invasive assessment is not limited by the factors that confound echocardiographic measurement mentioned above. In the presence of serial obstruction, an end hole catheter can be positioned above and below the point of interest and pressure gradients can be reassessed. In this scenario, it is possible to determine the site that contributes maximally to gradients—either the valve or the obstruction further down in the LVOT, thus facilitating accurate diagnosis.

Another advantage of invasive assessment is that the operators often perform coronary angiography prior to potentially inducing dobutamine stress. When there is no flow limiting coronary artery disease, higher doses of dobutamine (up to 40 μg/kg body weight) can be used to obtain a conclusive result. When there is associated significant coronary artery disease, high dose dobutamine (>30 μg/kg body weight) can result in a "biphasic response," further reducing blood flow across the aortic valve, thus confounding results. This is one of the main reasons why a low dose dobutamine is recommended when doing a DSE. In the cardiac catherization laboratory however, any significant coronary artery disease can be treated percutaneously before escalating to higher doses of dobutamine to diagnose LFLG severe AS.

The disadvantage of invasive assessment is the potential complications of cardiac catheterization, especially when crossing the heavily calcified aortic valve; in particular stroke. In the presence of a small aortic root, the phenomenon of "pressure recovery" may confound gradients by increasing aortic pressure and under estimating transvalvular pressure gradients.

The diagnosis of LFLG severe aortic stenosis requires a systematic approach with a series of tests. **Figure 16** summarizes an algorithm for assessment of low flow low gradient aortic stenosis.

4. Prognosis and management

The importance of establishing the diagnosis of LFLG severe AS is reflected in its differing prognosis to high gradient severe AS. Not only are the outcomes with conservative management worse in LFLG AS, studies have also suggested poorer outcomes following intervention.

4.1 "Classical" low flow low gradient severe AS with reduced left ventricular ejection fraction: (stage D2)

Among the subgroups of severe AS, classical LFLG AS has the worst clinical outcome. With medical management the 2-year survival is approximately 40–60%. Thirty-day mortality of SAVR is high depending on the presence or absence of flow reserve (8–33%) [8, 9, 12, 13, 29]. However, if patients survive SAVR, there is a prognostic benefit compared to medical therapy. There is limited head to head randomized data comparing SAVR and TAVR in patients with LFLG severe AS. There are few studies that suggest that TAVR leads to better and faster LV function recovery compared to SAVR [45, 46]. It is well known that TAVR, especially with supra-annular valves leads to less patient prosthesis mismatch, which is an independent predictor of worse outcomes [46], especially in patients with reduced LV ejection fraction. In patients with no flow reserve who represent the highest risk subgroup, TAVR may have a definite survival benefit over SAVR. Thought the PARTNER I trial conclusively proved the superiority of TAVR to medical management and similar outcomes to SAVR [47], patients with no LV flow reserve as well as those with very low LVEF were excluded. More randomized studies are needed to confirm the superiority of TAVR over SAVR in patients with classical LFLG severe AS (stage D2).

The heart team plays the central role in selecting the most appropriate modality of treatment, i.e., TAVR versus SAVR versus medical management (**Figure 17**).

A comprehensive risk stratification algorithm that takes into consideration risk scores (STS), frailty indices, major organ compromise and procedure specific impediments is used by the heart team to risk stratify the patient. Ideally the risk stratification process may also take into consideration specific factors that are not mentioned in the guidelines. These include preoperative NHYA class >III, low trans-aortic gradient (<20 mmHg), absence of flow reserve and reduced global longitudinal strain. A reduced global longitudinal strain, by itself suggests high risk, independent of risk scores (STS/Euroscore) [8, 9, 12].

Palliative balloon aortic valvuloplasty and medical management should be considered in patients with an expected life expectancy <1 year (**Figure 17**). In patients with classical LFLG severe AS with prohibitive and high surgical risk TAVR is recommended. In patients with intermediate surgical risk, SAVR or TAVR may be considered depending heart team evaluation; depending on other factors such as frailty, major organ compromise and procedure specific impediments (hostile chest in case of SAVR or vascular access route for TAVR).

4.2 Paradoxical low flow low gradient severe AS with preserved ejection fraction (stage D3)

Patients with paradoxical LFLG AS fare better than patients with classical LFLG AS [5, 18, 48]. The PARTNER I cohort B is the only randomized trial that reports better survival after TAVR compared to medical management [47], all other studies

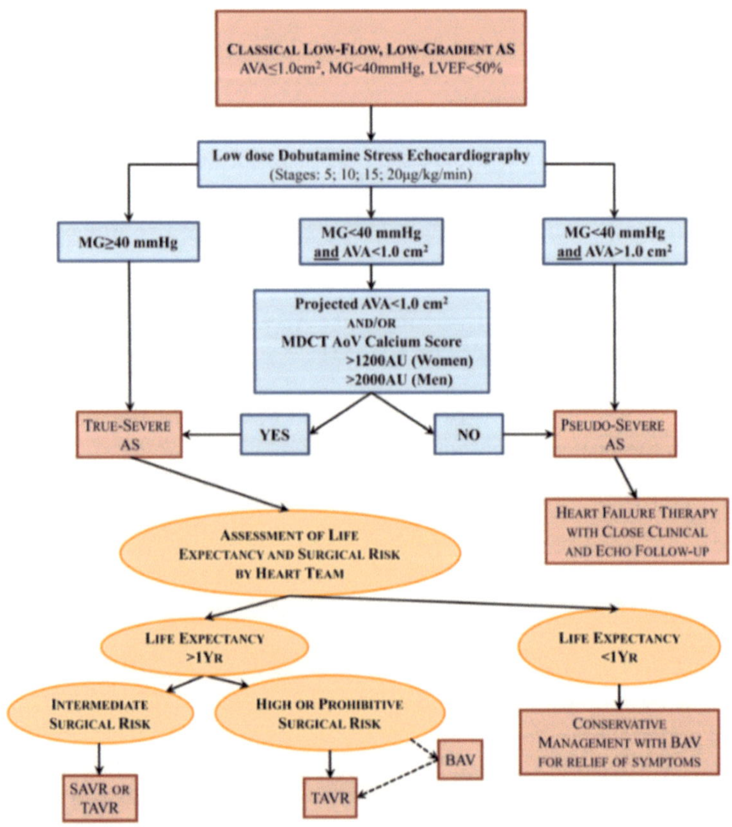

Figure 17.
Algorithm for the management of classical (reduced left ventricular ejection fraction) low-flow, low-gradient aortic stenosis. AoV, aortic valve; BAV, balloon aortic valvuloplasty; MDCT, multi-detector computed tomography; SAVR, surgical aortic valve replacement; TAVR, transcatheter aortic valve replacement. Reproduced with permission from Clavel et al. [32].

being observational. AVR reduces mortality by 57% in patients with paradoxical LFLG AS [49].

LVEF is a relatively poor and misleading parameter in assessing LV function especially in paradoxical LFLG AS. Higher degree of myocardial fibrosis documented either by cardiac magnetic resonance imaging or global longitudinal strain are independent risk factors for mortality in patients with paradoxical LFLG AS [50, 51].

The role of plasma brain natriuretic peptide (BNP) in risk stratification of patients with paradoxical LFLG AS is unclear [30]. Owing to significant LV concentric remodeling and small LV cavities, the LV wall stress may even be normal, thus the extent of myocardial stretch and release of BNP may not accurately reflect the severity of impairment of myocardial structure/function in these patients.

A systematic heart team approach is recommended to optimize outcomes (**Figure 18**). Aortic valve replacement should be considered in symptomatic patients with paradoxical LFLG and true severe AS. TAVR may be superior to SAVR in patients with paradoxical LFLG AS [47]. Certain factors intrinsic to patients with paradoxical LFLG AS pose higher surgical risks compared to patients with high gradient AS. These include higher prevalence in female sex, older age, systemic hypertension, atrial fibrillation, restrictive LV physiology and smaller aortic annulus that predisposes to patient prosthesis mismatch [52–54]. TAVR was associated

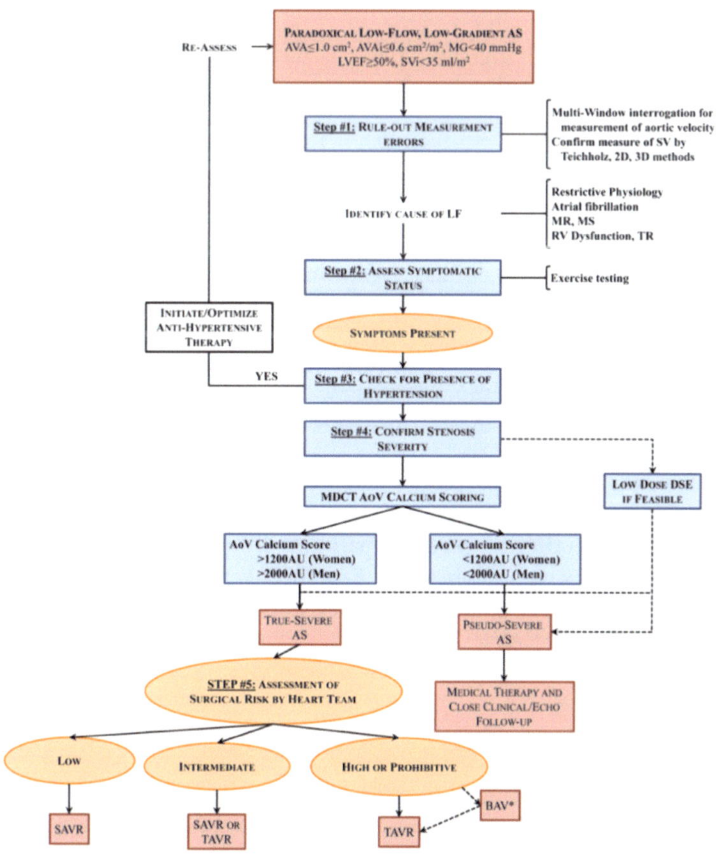

Figure 18.
Algorithm for the management of paradoxical (preserved left ventricular ejection fraction) low-flow, low-gradient aortic stenosis. AVAi, indexed aortic valve area; MR, mitral regurgitation; MS, mitral stenosis; TR, tricuspid regurgitation. Reproduced with permission from Clavel et al. [32].

with better 1-year survival compared with SAVR in patients with paradoxical LFLG AS in the PARTNER-I Cohort A trial. Further studies are needed to confirm the potential superiority of TAVR versus SAVR in this subset of patients.

5. Role of diagnostic balloon aortic valvuloplasty

In 1986, Cribier et al. [55] first described balloon aortic valvuloplasty (BAV) as a treatment strategy for patients with symptomatic severe AS presenting in cardiogenic shock, or who were deemed too high risk for conventional SAVR. Due to procedural complications, high incidence of restenosis within 6 months, lack of sustained clinical and hemodynamic benefit, BAV was not routinely performed. Furthermore, mortality rates within a year of BAV was similar to others with severe AS who were managed conservatively [56].

Table 1 lists the current status of BAV according to major guidelines. BAV has a class IIb recommendation for use as a bridge therapy to TAVR or SAVR in hemodynamically unstable patients at high risk for surgery. In the European guidelines (2017) BAV is recommended as a palliative measure in patients not suitable for TAVR or SAVR and in patients with symptomatic severe AS who require urgent noncardiac surgery. The American Heart Association (AHA)/American College of Cardiology (ACC) guidelines (2014) are similar to the European guidelines except they do not recommend the use of BAV as a palliative procedure nor its use in patients undergoing urgent non-cardiac surgery. However it does acknowledge that some patients report an improvement in their symptoms post BAV. The role of BAV as bridge to decision in high-risk patients has been supported by a number of studies [57]. The rationale behind such a strategy is listed below.

i. BAV helps to choose the best therapeutic option for each patient; avoiding expensive or high risk intervention for patients who may not have prognostic benefit from definitive treatment of AS.

ii. BAV may be utilized to palliate symptoms and reduce operative risk while awaiting TAVR or SAVR.

iii. BAV may be used as a diagnostic procedure especially in patients with concomitant severe pulmonary disease. The improvement in symptom status post BAV can attribute dyspnea to severe AS rather than lung disease alone.

iv. DSE is used to assess contractile reserve in patients with severe AS. It helps in diagnosis and predicting perioperative mortality but cannot predict LV function recovery. In this subgroup of patients, LV function can be reassessed after 4–8 weeks after "diagnostic" BAV. Recovery of LV function post BAV is a good indicator of contractile reserve and predicts sustained LV function improvement post SAVR/TAVR [58].

v. It has been demonstrated that nearly 50% of patients with severe AS and coexistent mitral regurgitation (MR) showed a reduction in the magnitude of MR after BAV [59]. A similar reduction is also seen with pulmonary artery systolic pressure [60]. BAV therefore negates the need for multiple valve intervention and reduces the overall the risk of SAVR.

vi. BAV may be used as a palliative procedure in patients with serious comorbidities, frailty, cognitive alteration, severe lung disease or life expectancy less than a year.

Indication for BAV in severe symptomatic aortic stenosis	ESC (2017)	ACC/AHA (2014)
As bridge therapy for all patients undergoing TAVI or AVR	✗	✓
As bridge therapy for haemodynamically unstable patients undergoing TAVI or AVR	✓	✓
For patients requiring urgent non-non-cardiac surgery	✓	✗
Palliative BAV for symptom benefit	✓	✗

Table 1.
Summary of ESC and ACC/AHA guidelines for the role of BAV in managing symptomatic severe AS.

6. Conclusion

Clinicians should be mindful that patients with symptomatic severe AS may well have low flow and thereby low gradient. Occasionally symptoms may represent severity of underlying heart failure rather than the severity of AS. Established minimally invasive trans-catheter therapies, although has improved associated morbidities of SAVR for intermediate and high-risk patients, it is important that treatment is directed to those who will benefit the most. Accurate diagnosis of severe AS is important as treatment modalities and its timing can offer prognostic benefits in the immediate and long term.

Conflict of interest

Faeez Mohamad Ali and Vindhya Wilson—no conflict of interest.
Rajesh Nair—proctor for Medtronic.

Author details

Faeez Mohamad Ali[1], Vindhya Wilson[2] and Rajesh Nair[1]*

1 Waikato Hospital, Hamilton, New Zealand

2 Nelson Hospital, New Zealand

*Address all correspondence to: drrnair@gmail.com

References

[1] Clavel MA, Burwash IG, Pibarot P. Cardiac imaging for assessing low-gradient severe aortic stenosis. JACC: Cardiovascular Imaging. 2017;**10**(2):185-202

[2] Nishimura RA, Otto CM, Bonow RO, Carabello BA, Erwin JP 3rd, Guyton RA, et al. 2014 AHA/ACC guideline for the management of patients with valvular heart disease: A report of the American College of Cardiology/ American Heart Association Task Force on Practice Guidelines. Journal of the American College of Cardiology. 2014;**63**(22):e57-e185

[3] Baumgartner H, Hung J, Bermejo J, Chambers JB, Evangelista A, Griffin BP, et al. Echocardiographic assessment of valve stenosis: EAE/ASE recommendations for clinical practice. Journal of the American Society of Echocardiography. 2009;**22**(1):1-23

[4] Vahanian A, Alfieri O, Andreotti F, Antunes MJ, Barón-Esquivias G, Baumgartner H, et al. Guidelines on the management of valvular heart disease (version 2012). Joint Task Force on the Management of Valvular Heart Disease of the European Society of Cardiology (ESC); European Association for Cardio Thoracic Surgery (EACTS). European Heart Journal. 2012;**33**(19):2451-2496

[5] Hachicha Z, Dumesnil JG, Bogaty P, Pibarot P. Paradoxical low flow, low gradient severe aortic stenosis despite preserved ejection fraction is associated with higher afterload and reduced survival. Circulation. 2007;**115**(22):2856-2864

[6] Berthelot-Richer M, Pibarot P, Capoulade R, Dumesnil JG, Dahou A, Thebault C, et al. Discordant grading of aortic stenosis severity: Echocardiographic predictors of survival benefit associated with aortic valve replacement. JACC: Cardiovascular Imaging. 2016;**9**(7):797-805

[7] Minners J, Allgeier M, Gohlke-Baerwolf C, Kienzle RP, Neumann FJ, Jander N. Inconsistent grading of aortic valve stenosis by current guidelines: Haemodynamic studies in patients with apparently normal left ventricular function. Heart. 2010;**96**(18):1463-1468

[8] Connolly HM, Oh JK, Schaff HV, Roger VL, Osborn SL, Hodge DO, et al. Severe aortic stenosis with low transvalvular gradient and severe left ventricular dysfunction. Result of aortic valve replacement in 52 patients. Circulation. 2000;**101**(16):1940-1946

[9] Monin JL, Quéré JP, Monchi M, Petit H, Baleynaud S, Chauvel C, et al. Low-gradient aortic stenosis: Operative risk stratification and predictors for long term outcome: A multicenter study using dobutamine stress hemodynamics. Circulation. 2003;**108**(3):319-324

[10] Brogan WC 3rd, Grayburn PA, Lange RA, Hillis LD. Prognosis after valve replacement in patients with severe aortic stenosis and a low transvalvular pressure gradient. Journal of the American College of Cardiology. 1993;**21**(7):1657-1660

[11] Levy F, Laurent M, Monin JL, Maillet JM, Pasquet A, Le Tourneau T, et al. Aortic valve replacement for low-flow/low-gradient aortic stenosis: Operative risk stratification and long term outcome: A European multicenter study. Journal of the American College of Cardiology. 2008;**51**(15):1466-1472

[12] Tribouilloy C, Lévy F, Rusinaru D, Guéret P, Petit-Eisenmann H, Baleynaud S, et al. Outcome after aortic valve replacement for low-flow/ low-gradient aortic stenosis without contractile reserve on dobutamine

stress echocardiography. Journal of the American College of Cardiology. 2009;**53**(20):1865-1873

[13] Clavel MA, Fuchs C, Burwash IG, Mundigler G, Dumesnil JG, Baumgartner H, et al. Predictors of outcomes in low-flow, low-gradient aortic stenosis: Results of the multicenter TOPAS study. Circulation. 2008;**118**(14 Suppl):S234-S242

[14] Otto CM, Burwash IG, Legget ME, Munt BI, Fujioka M, Healy NL, et al. Prospective study of asymptomatic valvular aortic stenosis. Clinical, echocardiographic, and exercise predictors of outcome. Circulation. 1997;**95**(9):2262-2270

[15] Rosenhek R, Zilberszac R, Schemper M, Czerny M, Mundigler G, Graf S, et al. Natural history of very severe aortic stenosis. Circulation. 2010;**121**(1):151-156

[16] Ross J Jr, Braunwald E. Aortic stenosis. Circulation. 1968;**38** (1 Suppl):61-67

[17] Dumesnil JG, Pibarot P, Carabello B. Paradoxical low flow and/or low gradient severe aortic stenosis despite preserved left ventricular ejection fraction: Implications for diagnosis and treatment. European Heart Journal. 2010;**31**(3):281-289

[18] Lancellotti P, Magne J, Donal E, Davin L, O'Connor K, Rosca M, et al. Clinical outcome in asymptomatic severe aortic stenosis. Insights from the new proposed aortic stenosis grading classification. Journal of the American College of Cardiology. 2012;**59**(3):235-243

[19] Baumgartner H, Hung J, Bermejo J, Chambers JB, Evangelista A, Griffin BP, et al. EAE/ASE. Echocardiographic assessment of valve stenosis: EAE/ASE recommendations for clinical practice. European Journal of Echocardiography. 2009;**10**(1):1-25

[20] Fougères E, Tribouilloy C, Monchi M, Petit-Eisenmann H, Baleynaud S, Pasquet A, et al. Outcomes of pseudo-severe aortic stenosis under conservative treatment. European Heart Journal. 2012;**33**(19):2426-2433

[21] Clavel MA, Burwash IG, Mundigler G, Dumesnil JG, Baumgartner H, Bergler-Klein J, et al. Validation of conventional and simplified methods to calculate projected valve area at normal flow rate in patients with low flow, low gradient aortic stenosis: The multicenter TOPAS (True or Pseudo-Severe Aortic Stenosis) study. Journal of the American Society of Echocardiography. 2010;**23**(4):380-386

[22] Samad Z, Vora AN, Dunning A, Schulte PJ, Shaw LK, Al-Enezi F, et al. Aortic valve surgery and survival in patients with moderate or severe aortic stenosis and left ventricular dysfunction. European Heart Journal. 2016;**37**(28):2276-2286

[23] Thaden JJ, Nkomo VT, Lee KJ, Oh JK. Doppler imaging in aortic stenosis: The importance of the nonapical imaging windows to determine severity in a contemporary cohort. Journal of the American Society of Echocardiography. 2015;**28**(7):780-785

[24] Skjaerpe T, Hegrenaes L, Hatle L. Noninvasive estimation of valve area in patients with aortic stenosis by Doppler ultrasound and two dimensional echocardiography. Circulation. 1985;**72**(4):810-818

[25] LaBounty TM, Miyasaka R, Chetcuti S, Grossman PM, Deeb GM, Patel HJ, et al. Annulus instead of LVOT diameter improves agreement between echocardiography effective orifice area and invasive aortic valve area. JACC: Cardiovascular Imaging. 2014;**7**(10):1065-1066

[26] deFilippi CR, Willett DL, Brickner ME, Appleton CP, Yancy

CW, Eichhorn EJ, et al. Usefulness of dobutamine echocardiography in distinguishing severe from nonsevere valvular aortic stenosis in patients with depressed left ventricular function and low transvalvular gradients. The American Journal of Cardiology. 1995;**75**(2):191-194

[27] Nishimura RA, Grantham JA, Connolly HM, Schaff HV, Higano ST, Holmes DR Jr. Low-output, low-gradient aortic stenosis in patients with depressed left ventricular systolic function: The clinical utility of the dobutamine challenge in the catheterization laboratory. Circulation. 2002;**106**(7):809-813

[28] Picano E, Pibarot P, Lancellotti P, Monin JL, Bonow RO. The emerging role of exercise testing and stress echocardiography in valvular heart disease. Journal of the American College of Cardiology. 2009;**54**(24):2251-2260

[29] Quere JP, Monin JL, Levy F, Petit H, Baleynaud S, Chauvel C, et al. Influence of preoperative left ventricular contractile reserve on postoperative ejection fraction in low-gradient aortic stenosis. Circulation. 2006;**113**(14):1738-1744

[30] Bergler-Klein J, Mundigler G, Pibarot P, Burwash IG, Dumesnil JG, Blais C, et al. B-type natriuretic peptide in low-flow, low-gradient aortic stenosis: Relationship to hemodynamics and clinical outcome. Circulation. 2007;**115**(22):2848-2855

[31] Blais C, Burwash IG, Mundigler G, Dumesnil JG, Loho N, Rader F, et al. Projected valve area at normal flow rate improves the assessment of stenosis severity in patients with low flow, low-gradient aortic stenosis: The multicenter TOPAS (Truly or Pseudo-Severe Aortic Stenosis) study. Circulation. 2006;**113**(5):711-721

[32] Clavel M-A, Magne J, Pibarot P. Low-gradient aortic stenosis. European Heart Journal. 2016;**37**(34):2645-2657

[33] Burwash IG, Lortie M, Pibarot P, de Kemp RA, Graf S, Mundigler G, et al. Myocardial blood flow in patients with low flow, low gradient aortic stenosis: Differences between true and pseudo-severe aortic stenosis. Results from the multicenter TOPAS (Truly or Pseudo-Severe Aortic Stenosis) study. Heart. 2008;**94**(12):1627-1633

[34] Clavel MA, Messika-Zeitoun D, Pibarot P, Aggarwal SR, Malouf J, Araoz PA, et al. The complex nature of discordant severe calcified aortic valve disease grading: New insights from combined Doppler echocardiographic and computed tomographic study. Journal of the American College of Cardiology. 2013;**62**(24):2329-2338

[35] Agatston AS, Janowitz WR, Hildner FJ, Zusmer NR, Viamonte M Jr, Detrano R. Quantification of coronary artery calcium using ultrafast computed tomography. Journal of the American College of Cardiology. 1990;**15**(4):827-832

[36] Cueff C, Serfaty JM, Cimadevilla C, Laissy JP, Himbert D, Tubach F, et al. Measurement of aortic valve calcification using multislice computed tomography: Correlation with haemodynamic severity of aortic stenosis and clinical implication for patients with low ejection fraction. Heart. 2011;**97**(9):721-726

[37] Clavel MA, Pibarot P, Messika-Zeitoun D, Capoulade R, Malouf J, Aggarval S, et al. Impact of aortic valve calcification, as measured by MDCT, on survival in patients with aortic stenosis: Results of an international registry study. Journal of the American College of Cardiology. 2014;**64**(12):1202-1213

[38] Aggarwal SR, Clavel MA, Messika-Zeitoun D, Cueff C, Malouf J, Araoz PA, et al. Sex differences in aortic valve

calcification measured by multidetector computed tomography in aortic stenosis. Circulation. Cardiovascular Imaging. 2013;**6**(1):40-47

[39] Shen M, Tastet L, Capoulade R, Larose É, Bédard É, Arsenault M, et al. Effect of age and aortic valve anatomy on calcification and haemodynamic severity of aortic stenosis. Heart. 2017;**103**(1):32-39

[40] Jilaihawi H, Doctor N, Kashif M, Chakravarty T, Rafique A, Makar M, et al. Aortic annular sizing for transcatheter aortic valve replacement using cross sectional 2-dimensional transesophageal echocardiography. Journal of the American College of Cardiology. 2013;**61**(9):908-916

[41] Chin CW, Khaw HJ, Luo E, Tan S, White AC, Newby DE, et al. Echocardiography underestimates stroke volume and aortic valve area: Implications for patients with small area low-gradient aortic stenosis. The Canadian Journal of Cardiology. 2014;**30**(9):1064-1072

[42] Khalique OK, Kodali SK, Paradis JM, Nazif TM, Williams MR, Einstein AJ, et al. Aortic annular sizing using a novel 3-dimensional echocardiographic method: Use and comparison with cardiac computed tomography. Circulation. Cardiovascular Imaging. 2014;**7**(1):155-163

[43] Clavel MA, Malouf J, Messika-Zeitoun D, Araoz PA, Michelena HI, Enriquez-Sarano M. Aortic valve area calculation in aortic stenosis by CT and Doppler echocardiography. JACC: Cardiovascular Imaging. 2015;**8**(3):248-257

[44] Kamperidis V, van Rosendael PJ, Katsanos S, van der Kley F, Regeer M, Al Amri I, et al. Low gradient severe aortic stenosis with preserved ejection fraction: Reclassification of severity by fusion of Doppler and computed tomographic data. European Heart Journal. 2015;**36**(31):2087-2096

[45] Clavel MA, Webb JG, Rodés-Cabau J, Masson JB, Dumont E, De Larochellière R, et al. Comparison between transcatheter and surgical prosthetic valve implantation in patients with severe aortic stenosis and reduced left ventricular ejection fraction. Circulation. 2010;**122**(19):1928-1936

[46] Ben-Dor I, Maluenda G, Iyasu GD, Laynez-Carnicero A, Hauville C, Torguson R, et al. Comparison of outcome of higher versus lower transvalvular gradients in patients with severe aortic stenosis and low (<40%) left ventricular ejection fraction. The American Journal of Cardiology. 2012;**109**(7):1031-1037

[47] Herrmann HC, Pibarot P, Hueter I, Gertz ZM, Stewart WJ, Kapadia S, et al. Predictors of mortality and outcomes of therapy in low-flow severe aortic stenosis: A Placement of Aortic Transcatheter Valves (PARTNER) trial analysis. Circulation. 2013;**127**(23):2316-2326

[48] Eleid MF, Sorajja P, Michelena HI, Malouf JF, Scott CG, Pellikka PA. Flow-gradient patterns in severe aortic stenosis with preserved ejection fraction: Clinical characteristics and predictors of survival. Circulation. 2013;**128**(16):1781-1789

[49] Dayan V, Vignolo G, Magne J, Clavel MA, Mohty D, Pibarot P. Outcome and impact of aortic valve replacement in patients with preserved LV ejection fraction and low gradient aortic stenosis: A meta-analysis. Journal of the American College of Cardiology. 2015;**66**(23):2594-2603

[50] Herrmann S, Störk S, Niemann M, Lange V, Strotmann JM, Frantz S, et al. Low-gradient aortic valve stenosis: Myocardial fibrosis and its influence on function and outcome. Journal of

the American College of Cardiology. 2011;**58**(4):402-412

[51] Le Ven F, Freeman M, Webb J, Clavel MA, Wheeler M, Dumont É, et al. Impact of low flow on the outcome of high risk patients undergoing transcatheter aortic valve replacement. Journal of the American College of Cardiology. 2013;**62**(9):782-788

[52] Mohty D, Magne J, Deltreuil M, Aboyans V, Echahidi N, Cassat C, et al. Outcome and impact of surgery in paradoxical low-flow, low-gradient severe aortic stenosis and preserved left ventricular ejection fraction: A cardiac catheterization study. Circulation. 2013;**128**(11 Suppl 1):S235-S242

[53] Clavel MA, Berthelot-Richer M, Le Ven F, Capoulade R, Dahou A, Dumesnil JG, et al. Impact of classic and paradoxical low flow on survival after aortic valve replacement for severe aortic stenosis. Journal of the American College of Cardiology. 2015;**65**(7):645-653

[54] Mohty D, Boulogne C, Magne J, Pibarot P, Echahidi N, Cornu E, et al. Prevalence and long term outcome of aortic prosthesis-patient mismatch in patients with paradoxical low-flow severe aortic stenosis. Circulation. 2014;**130**(11 Suppl 1):S25-S31

[55] Cribier A, Savin T, Saoudi N, et al. Percutaneous transluminal aortic valvuloplasty using a balloon catheter. A new therapeutic option in aortic stenosis in the elderly. Arch Mal Coeur Vaiss. 1986;**79**:1678-1686

[56] Ben-Dor I, Pichard AD, Satler LF, Goldstein SA, Syed AI, Gaglia MA Jr, et al. Complications and outcome of balloon aortic valvuloplasty in high-risk or inoperable patients. JACC. Cardiovascular Interventions. 2010;**3**(11):1150-1156

[57] Saia F, Moretti C, Dall'Ara G, Ciuca C, Taglieri N, Berardini A, et al. Balloon aortic valvuloplasty as a bridge-to-decision in high risk patients with aortic stenosis: A new paradigm for the heart team decision making. Journal of Geriatric Cardiology. 2016;**13**(6):475-482

[58] Berland J, Cribier A, Savin T, Lefebvre E, Koning R, Letac B. Percutaneous balloon valvuloplasty in patients with severe aortic stenosis and low ejection fraction. Immediate results and 1-year follow-up. Circulation. 1989;**79**(6):1189-1196

[59] Maluenda G, Ben-Dor I, Laynez-Carnicero A, Barbash IM, Sardi G, Gaglia MA Jr, et al. Changes in mitral regurgitation after balloon aortic valvuloplasty. The American Journal of Cardiology. 2011;**108**(12):1777-1782

[60] Ben-Dor I, Goldstein SA, Pichard AD, Satler LF, Maluenda G, Li Y, et al. Clinical profile, prognostic implication, and response to treatment of pulmonary hypertension in patients with severe aortic stenosis. The American Journal of Cardiology. 2011;**107**(7):1046-1051

Chapter 3

Current Management of Severe Aortic Stenosis in Intermediate Risk Patients

Omer Leal, Diego Sanchez-Valenzuela and Juan Bustamante-Munguira

Abstract

The management of aortic stenosis has improved and evolved to a reduction in surgical aggression. Nowadays, patients with intermediate risk are in the frontier of transcatheter aortic valve implantation (TAVI) and aortic valve replacement (AVR). Our goal is to update the treatment of severe aortic stenosis in those patients through a research of the recent literature, in order to analyze the current treatment options and their results. This cohort of patients has two therapeutic options, surgical AVR or TAVI, and the decision pathway goes through the accurate interpretation of all data by the Heart Team. It is clear that both strategies will be the cornerstones in the modern AVR era, but the situations in which to apply each strategy have not yet been clearly delineated. More studies are needed to compare TAVI and miniAVR in low- and intermediate-risk patients. However, the current practice guidelines give a good pathway to choose the adequate therapeutic option in each individual case.

Keywords: aortic stenosis, aortic stenosis surgery, aortic stenosis management, aortic stenosis open heart surgery, aortic stenosis treatment, aortic stenosis valve replacement, TAVR procedure, TAVR approaches, TAVR access sites, TAVR, TAVI

1. Introduction

Aortic stenosis is the most frequent valve disease leading to intervention in developed countries, either surgery or catheter, and its incidence increases due to the aging population [1].

The management of aortic stenosis has improved and evolved to a reduction in surgical aggression. Nowadays, the patients with intermediate risk are in the frontier of transcatheter aortic valve implantation (TAVI) and aortic valve replacement (AVR) and more than ever, the heart team has to be more accurate to choose between the different treatment options available, making the decision pathway more complex than a few year before. Our goal is to update the treatment of severe aortic stenosis in those patients where risk assessment scales indicate an intermediate risk. Here, we analyze the current treatment options and their results.

2. Etiology and natural history

Nowadays, degenerative calcific AS is the most common cause of AS in adults at older ages and represents the leading cause for aortic valve intervention [2–4]. In the other hand, bicuspid aortic valve affects 2% of the population and represents the most common indication for intervention at younger patients [5].

The development of symptoms identifies a paramount point in the natural history of AS, and the interval from the onset of symptoms to the time of death is approximately 2 years in patients with heart failure, 3 years in those with syncope, and 5 years in those with angina, with a high risk of sudden death [6].

3. Evaluation and severity classification of aortic stenosis

Careful exploration for the presence of symptoms (shortness of breath on exertion, angina, dizziness, or syncope) is very important for right patient management. The characteristic systolic murmur draws attention and guides further diagnostic work in the right direction.

Echocardiography is the key diagnostic tool [7]. It discriminates the degree of valve calcification, LV function, and wall thickness; helps to identify other associated valve diseases or aortic pathology; and provides prognostic information. The severity of the stenotic lesion can be defined with Doppler echocardiographic measurements. Transoesophageal echocardiography (TOE) provides additional evaluation of concomitant mitral valve abnormalities, and become useful when transthoracic visualization is poor [8]. TOE has gained importance in the assessment and intraprocedure guidance and after TAVI or surgical interventions.

Three-dimensional TOE offers a more detailed examination of valve anatomy than two-dimensional echocardiography and is useful for the assessment and planning of complex valve problems [8]. AS severity could be graded on the basis of a variety of hemodynamic and natural history data as shown in **Table 1**.

Multislice computed tomography (MSCT) and cardiac magnetic resonance (CMR) give additional data on the assessment of the ascending aorta when it is enlarged or to quantifying the valve area, coronary calcification, size and shape of the aortic valve annulus, and its distance to the coronary ostia, which aids in evaluation and prognosis. It is essential to evaluate the feasibility of the various access routes for TAVI, as this provides information on minimal luminal diameters, atherosclerotic plaque burden, the presence of aneurysms or thrombi, etc. [8]. MSCT plays an important role in the diagnostic work-up before transcatheter aortic valve implantation. The risk of radiation exposure—and of renal failure due to contrast injection—should, however, be taken into consideration.

Peak velocity (m/s)	≥4
Mean gradient (mmHg)	≥40
Indexed AVA (cm^2/m^2)	<0.6
AVA (cm^2)	<1
Velocity ratio	<0.25

Based on the recommendations on the echocardiographic assessment of aortic valve stenosis: a focused update from the European Association of Cardiovascular Imaging and the American Society of Echocardiography [9].

Table 1.
Severe aortic stenosis measurement by echocardiography. The definitions apply only in the presence of normal flow conditions.

In patients with inadequate echocardiographic quality or discrepant results, CMR should be used to assess the severity of valvular lesions and to assess ventricular volumes and systolic function [8].

In physically active patients, an **exercise testing** could be recommended for unmasking symptoms and for risk stratification of asymptomatic patients [10]. Also, exercise stress echocardiography may give prognostic information in asymptomatic severe aortic stenosis [10, 11]. In some patients, it may be necessary to proceed with cardiac catheterization and coronary angiography at the time of initial evaluation [7].

Biomarkers. Several studies [12–15] report that biomarkers such as B-type natriuretic peptide (BNP) have been shown to be related to functional class and prognosis, particularly in AS and MR. Natriuretic peptides have been shown to predict symptom-free survival and outcome in normal- and low-flow severe AS and may be useful in asymptomatic patients, helping to discriminate those patients who can benefit from an early intervention [13–15]. In fact, in the last ESC/EACTS guidelines for the management of valvular heart disease, natriuretic peptides may be of value for risk stratification and timing of intervention, particularly in asymptomatic patients ("markedly elevated BNP levels (>threefold age- and sex-corrected normal range) confirmed by repeated measurements without other explanations") [8].

4. Indications for intervention

Here, we have to take notice of the patient's status in order to choose the type of intervention and the correct timing of it. **Early valve intervention should be strongly recommended in all symptomatic patients with severe AS, because it is the only effective treatment.** "As long as the mean gradient remains >40 mmHg, there is virtually no lower ejection fraction limit for intervention, whether surgery or TAVI" [8].

However, patients with severe comorbidities indicating a survival of <1 year and patients in whom is unlikely that the intervention will improve quality of life or survival should be excluded from further interventions.

Asymptomatic patients. There is some disagreement about the optimal timing of surgery in asymptomatic patients, and the decision to operate on this kind of patient requires careful weighing of the benefits against the risks.

The available studies do not provide convincing data to support the general recommendation of early SAVR, even in patients with asymptomatic and very severe aortic stenosis, and TAVI is not recommended in asymptomatic patients [7, 8]. However, subclinical adverse remodeling can precede the development of symptoms and LV dysfunction [16]. Musa et al. performed cardiac magnetic resonance (CMR) in 674 patients who had severe AS and were scheduled for surgical or transcatheter AVR. Myocardial fibrosis (scar) demonstrated by late gadolinium enhancement (LGE) on CMR was common (51%). In a median follow-up of 3.6 years (interquartile range, 2.6–5.9 years), 21.5% of patients had died. In multivariable analysis, scar (LGE positivity) was independently associated with all-cause and cardiovascular mortality (hazard ratios, 2.39 and 3.14, respectively). The elevated mortality was independent of whether the patients underwent surgical or transcatheter AVR and was similar in patients with infarct and noninfarct scar patterns. These findings raise the possibility that adverse remodeling has irreversible effects before symptoms develop: We may be waiting too long to treat these patients. The authors suggest that physicians might use scar burden to optimize the timing of intervention, a hypothesis currently being evaluated in a randomized trial (EVOLVED-AS) [16].

Early elective surgery is indicated in asymptomatic patients with [8]:

- depressed LV function not due to other causes and in patients who develop symptoms during exercise testing
- abnormal exercise test showing symptoms on exercise clearly related to aortic stenosis
- abnormal exercise test showing a decrease in blood pressure below baseline
- predictors of symptom development and adverse outcomes: clinical characteristics (older age, presence of atherosclerotic risk factors), echocardiographic parameters (valve calcification, peak aortic jet velocity, LVEF, rate of hemodynamic progression, increase in mean gradient >20 mmHg with exercise, excessive LV hypertrophy, abnormal longitudinal LV function, and pulmonary hypertension), and biomarkers (>threefold age- and sex-corrected normal range).
- When early elective surgery is considered in patients with normal exercise performance because of the presence of such outcome predictors, the operative risk should be low. In patients without predictive factors, watchful waiting appears safe and early surgery is unlikely to be beneficial.

An update of proposed management strategy for patients with severe AS by Leal et al. [17] is shown in **Figure 1**, based on the ESC/EACTS and ACC/ AHA guidelines on the management of valvular heart disease [8, 18].

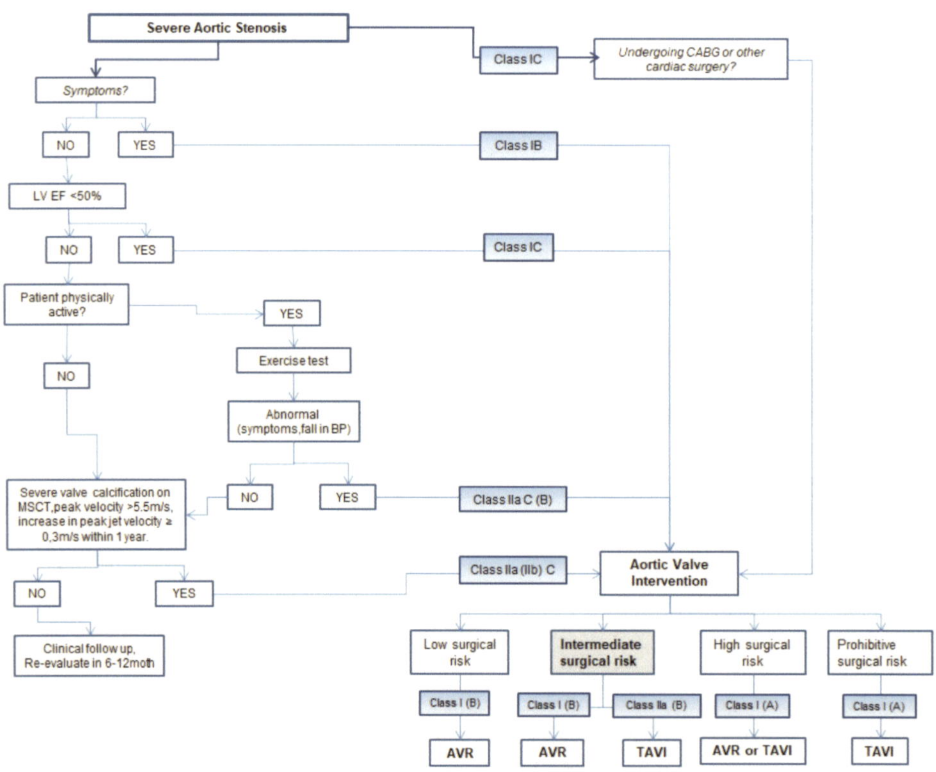

Figure 1.
Management of severe aortic stenosis [8, 17, 18]. ACC/AHA recommendations have been shown in parentheses.

5. Risk stratification

Risk stratification applies to any sort of intervention and is required for weighing the risk of intervention against the expected natural history of VHD as a basis for decision making [8]. Nowadays, the STS score and logistic EuroSCORE II are the most commonly used. **The EuroSCORE I** overestimates operative mortality and its calibration of risk is poor, and ***it should no longer be used to guide decision making,*** but it has been used in many TAVI studies/registries and may still be useful to identify the subgroups of patients for decision between intervention modalities and to predict 1-year mortality [8]. **The EuroSCORE II** and the **Society of Thoracic Surgeons (STS)** scores more accurately discriminate high- and low-risk surgical patients and show better calibration to predict postoperative outcome after valvular surgery [8]. Current models do not include some risk factors that may be particularly important in the prediction of outcomes, including frailty, pulmonary hypertension (PH), porcelain aorta, and the presence of hepatic dysfunction.

New scores have been developed to estimate the risk of 30-day mortality in patients undergoing TAVI, with better accuracy and discrimination, but not without certain limitations by a lack of consideration of frailty, disability, and cognitive function [19]. Examples of those are: FRANCE-2 risk score [20], the STS/ACC TVT registry predictive model [21], and the TAVR risk score based on data from the German aortic valve registry [22]. A new tool based on the STS/ACC TVT Registry™ is an application for from the STS/ACC TVT Registry™ an application for mobile devices and web, call **"TAVR in-hospital mortality Risk app"** [23], in order to inform physicians of the estimated risk of in-hospital mortality.

It remains essential not to rely on a single risk score figure when assessing patients or to determine unconditionally the indication and type of intervention.

The role of the heart team is essential to take all of these data into account and adopt a final decision on the best treatment strategy. It is important to take into account patient's life expectancy, expected quality of life, and patient preference, as well as local resources, in order to do a proper planning of intervention. There is a growing interest in the assessment of frailty, an overall marker of impairment of functional, cognitive, and nutritional status. Frailty is associated with increased morbidity and mortality after surgery and TAVI [24].

Finally, the patient and family should be thoroughly informed and assisted in their decision on the best treatment option.

Actual **AHA/ACC guideline** classifies patients with severe AS into ***four global risk categories***: [19].

1. Low risk: STS <4% with no frailty, no comorbidity, and no procedure-specific impediments.

2. **Intermediate risk: STS 4-8%** with no more than mild frailty or one major organ system compromise not to be improved postoperatively and minimal procedure-specific impediments.

3. High risk: STS >8%, or moderate-severe frailty, no more than two major organ systems compromise not to be improved postoperatively, or a possible procedure-specific impediment.

4. Prohibitive risk: preoperative risk of mortality and morbidity >50% at 1 year or ≥three major organ systems compromises not to be improved postoperatively or severe frailty or severe procedure-specific impediments.

Thus, the current **ESC/EACTS guidelines** for the management of valvular heart disease [8] consider ***two global risk categories***:

1. Low surgical risk (STS or EuroSCORE II < 4% or logistic EuroSCORE I < 10% and no other risk factors not included in these scores, such as frailty, porcelain aorta, and sequelae of chest radiation).

2. Increased surgical risk (STS or EuroSCORE II >4% or logistic EuroSCORE I > 10% or other risk factors not included in these scores such as frailty, porcelain aorta, and sequelae of chest radiation).

A resume of risk categories is shown in **Table 2**.

	Risk assessment tool		
Risk category	**STS score**	**EuroScore II**	**EuroScore**
Low risk	<4%	<4%	<10%
Intermediate risk	4–8%	>4–7%*	>10–20%*
High risk	>8%	>7*	>20%*
Prohibitive risk	>50%		

**ESC/EACTS guidelines consider two categories (low and increased surgical risk).*
Based on 2017 ACC Expert Consensus Decision Pathway for Transcatheter Aortic Valve Replacement in the Management of Adults with Aortic Stenosis and the 2017 ESC/EACTS Guidelines for the management of valvular heart disease [8, 19, 25].

Table 2.
Risk assessment tools.

In conclusion, the decision to proceed with AVR or TAVI requires careful weighing of the potential for improved symptoms and survival and the morbidity and mortality of surgery and should be made by the heart team according to the individual patient characteristics. Checklist for choice of therapeutic intervention option (**Table A1**) could be consulted and printed from the additional material, in order to provide aspects that should be considered for the individual decision, based on the current recommendation of de ESC/EACTS guidelines.

6. Interventional therapeutic options

6.1 Surgical approach

6.1.1 Conventional AVR

The conventional approach to AVR consists of a mid-line incision and full sternotomy, which provide a complete and comfortable access to the heart. Since it was first successfully carried out by Harken and Starr in 1960 [26, 27], there has been a continuous innovation in prosthetic technology and surgical techniques. All these collective efforts have resulted in improvements in both operative and long-term results [17]. Regardless of surgical approach, elected AVR is the gold standard for the treatment of severe AS. Several studies have shown short- and long-term outcomes, as well as improved quality of life. Operative outcomes following AVR were still improving in the past decade. Wu et al. [28], determined the economic value of the additional life given to patients undergoing AVR, and concluded that AVR is cost-effective for all ages, and still worthwhile in octogenarian and nonagenarian patients.

6.1.2 Minimally invasive surgical (MIS) approaches

Minimally invasive surgery aims to minimize the degree of surgical intrusiveness. Currently, there are several surgical approaches. The partial sternotomy and right anterior minithoracotomy are the most frequently used incisions for a minimally invasive approach to the aortic valve. The choice of interventional approach depends on the patient's anatomy as observed in preoperative imaging studies such as CT.

The "J" incision is the most widely used approach among the partial upper hemisternotomy approach (**Figure 2**). **Figure 3** shows the access view through right anterior minithoracotomy.

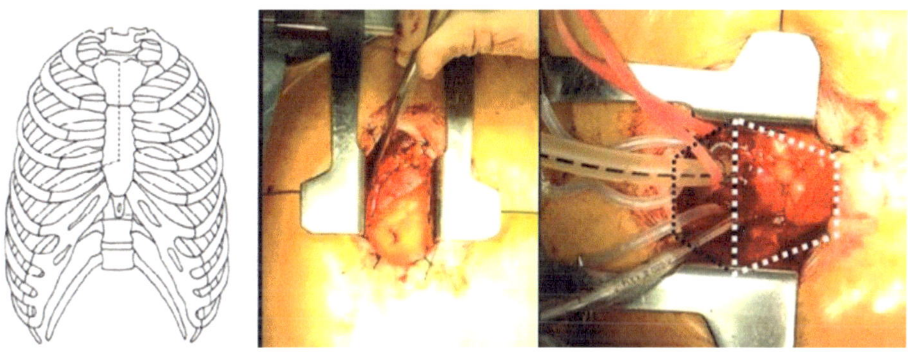

Figure 2.
Partial upper hemisternotomy approach. Operative field distribution from surgeon view [17].

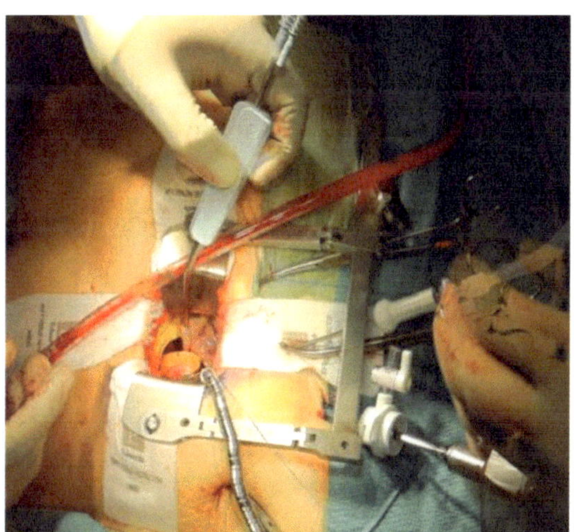

Figure 3.
Right anterior thoracotomy through 2 or 3° intercostal space [17].

6.1.2.1 Advantages and disadvantages of MIS approaches in aortic stenosis

Benefits have been observed in certain aspects such as:

- reduction in bleeding and use of hemoderivatives
- reduction in the pain perceived by the patient, which results in reduced consumption of analgesic [29–31]
- less respiratory complications such as atelectasis by maintaining the integrity of the thorax [32]
- better esthetic results, due to the reduced size of the surgical incisions and their relocation to less visible areas [33]
- reduction of the surgical wound infections [34]
- reduction on duration of hospitalization and time spent in intensive care units, which results on less expensive cost of the process.

A certain consensus exists around the benefits mentioned above. There is also a question of the impact of MIS on duration of surgery. There is disparity in the results found in the literature. Once the learning curve has been overcome, these times tend to equal out, and there is no significant difference to be observed between the different approaches.

6.1.3 Rapid deployment prostheses

Their use in association with MIS approaches, providing a reduction in surgical aggression in addition to the reduction in ECC and aortic clamping time. These designs have the common feature of being expandable, anchoring themselves to the aortic ring in a similar way to the devices used in TAVI. To date, there are two commercially available models: Perceval (LivaNova) and Intuity (Edwards Lifesciences). Those prostheses differ from each other in a few characteristics.

- **Perceval** (LivaNova): it is useful on patients in which a reduction in surgery time may have a paramount impact, or those where it is necessary to carry out mixed procedures [35, 36]. A recent multicenter study reports a reduction on mean crossclamp and cardiopulmonary bypass times, and a significant improvement in clinical status was observed postoperatively in the majority of patients [37]. The Perceval valve implantation could be easily performed by offering a significant reduction in crossclamping and CPB times compared with both the traditional valve prostheses and the other sutureless prostheses available on the market, even when performed via a minimally invasive approach [37]. It remains important for the continuation of the patient's follow-up, in order to provide further assessment of long-term valve performance [37].
- **Intuity** (Edwards Lifesciences): it is made by the conjunction between the Edwards Perimount bioprosthesis, the clinical and hemodynamic results of which are widely known, and the experience in the development of the Sapien transcatheter prosthesis. The mode of implantation for this prosthesis

allows the aortic clamping and extracorporeal circulation times to be reduced. Reports of early outcomes have shown an important reduction in aortic crossclamp and cardiopulmonary bypass (CPB) [38, 39]. These findings were confirmed in both the European TRITON [40] and the US TRANSFORM trials [41]. Even more important, these times were reduced significantly in combined cardiac procedures [38].

6.1.4 Transcatheter aortic valve implantation (TAVI)

TAVI was developed as an alternative to AVR in the very or extremely high-risk patient population, and its first implantation in man was performed by Cribier [42] in 2002. Since then, there has been a nonstop development of less invasive strategies with lower mortality, lower morbidity, and less invasiveness [43].

6.1.4.1 Implantation techniques

TAVI is currently carried out using two main approaches, **transfemoral** and **transapical**. If this is not feasible, then the other two main approaches could be used namely trans-axillary artery or transaortic approaches. It is, therefore, highly recommended to perform an adequate preoperative assessment of the degree of peripheral arterial disease through imaging studies such as CT.

6.1.4.2 TAVI results

The results of the PARTNER I Cohort A trial also have important implications. The primary endpoint of the trial was met, with TAVI found not to be inferior to aortic valve replacement for all-cause mortality at 1 year. Death at 30 days was lower than expected in both arms of the trial: TAVI mortality (3.4%) was the lowest reported in any series, despite an early generation device and limited previous operator experience. Aortic valve replacement mortality (6.5%) was lower than the expected operative mortality (11.8%). On 2015, the 5-year follow-up result of the PARTNER I trial was published [44]; they screened 3105 patients, of whom 699 were enrolled (348 assigned to TAVR, 351 assigned to SAVR). At 5 years, risk of death was 67·8% in the TAVR group compared with 62.4% in the SAVR group (hazard ratio 1.04, 95% CI 0.86–1.24; $p = 0.76$). They recorded no structural valve deterioration requiring surgical valve replacement in either group. Moderate or severe aortic regurgitation occurred in 40 (14%) of 280 patients in the TAVR group and two (1%) of 228 in the SAVR group ($p < 0.0001$), and was associated with the increased 5-year risk of mortality in the TAVR group [44].

7. Intermediate risk patients: who are they? And how do we have to manage them?

As we described before, currently AHA/ACC guideline for the management of patients with valvular heart disease [7, 19] defines the intermediate-risk patients as those who has an **STS 4–8%** with no more than mild frailty or one major organ system compromise not to be improved postoperatively and minimal procedure-specific impediments. In the other hand, the European guidelines define such patient as at "increased surgical risk" (STS or EuroSCORE II >4% or logistic EuroSCORE I > 10% or other risk factors not included in these scores such as frailty, porcelain aorta, and sequelae of chest radiation) [8].

This cohort of patients has two therapeutic options, surgical AVR or TAVI, and the decision pathway goes through the accurate interpretation of all data by the Heart Team.

Nowadays, increased operator experience and enhanced transcatheter valve systems have led to a worldwide trend to use TAVI in patients who are at low or intermediate risk [45]. This tendency has been evaluated in small observational studies, but since most patients who are currently recommended for surgery are at low or intermediate risk, the expansion of the use of TAVI demands more rigorous clinical-trial validation [46]. The intermediate-surgical-risk trials were approved comparing TAVI to surgery, with the balloon-expandable SAPIEN XT valve (PARTNER 2 trial) and the self-expandable CoreValve (SUrgical Replacement and Transcatheter Aortic Valve Implantation trial (SURTAVI trial)) [46, 47].

The PARTNER 2 trial [46] was a multicenter, randomized control trial conducted, which enrolled 2032 patients with severe symptomatic aortic stenosis and intermediate-surgical-risk, and randomized them in a 1:1 fashion across the TAVI arm and the surgical arm [48]. After 2 years, the all-cause mortality or disabling stroke was similar in the TAVI group and the SAVR group (19.3 vs. 21.1%, $p = 0.33$ and $p = 0.001$ for **noninferiority**). In the transfemoral access cohort, TAVI demonstrated a lower mortality and disabling stroke (hazard ratio = 0.79; 95% CI = 0.62–1.00; $p = 0.05$). TAVI resulted in larger aortic valve areas, lower rates of acute kidney injury, severe bleeding, and new-onset atrial fibrillation; SAVR resulted in fewer major vascular complications and less paravalvular aortic leak [49]. As a result of the PARTNER 2 trial, the current guideline from the American Heart Association and American College of Cardiology recommended TAVI as an alternative to surgery in patients at intermediate surgical risk [18, 48].

The SURTAVI trial [47] analyzes the self-expanding CoreValve in intermediate-risk patients and was a randomized, multicenter control trial, which recruited a total of 1746 patients [46]. The combined primary endpoint (all-cause mortality or disabling stroke) at 24 months was 12.6% in the TAVI group and 14.0% in the surgery group. Residual aortic regurgitation and need for pacemaker implantation were more frequent among TAVI patients. In the other hand, SAVR was associated with the higher rates of atrial fibrillation, acute kidney injury, and transfusion requirements. The TAVI resulted in lower mean gradients and larger aortic valve areas than surgery did. Structural valve deterioration at 24 months did not occur in either group. SURTAVI revealed that CoreValve TAVI was not inferior to surgery in patients with intermediate surgical risk [49].

Bicuspid aortic valves: the extreme and asymmetrical calcification noted with bicuspid valves can prevent adequate expansion of the valve frame of TAVI valves, affecting valve hemodynamics, and leading to higher aortic valve gradients and more paravalvular leaks [48].

Prostheses thrombosis: the Portico Re-sheathable Transcatheter Aortic Valve System U.S. Investigational Device Exemption (PORTICO IDE) study evaluates TAVI with either a Portico valve (St. Jude Medical) or a commercially available valve. Computed tomography (CT) was performed in a subgroup of patients to assess the stent frame of the implanted valve. A finding of reduced leaflet motion on CT in a patient who had had a stroke after TAVI and similar findings in an asymptomatic patient at one clinical site led to a closer look of this observation. Additional CT review by the core laboratory revealed that this finding was not isolated, which prompted a more extensive investigation. This findings encourage to create two registries to evaluate the prostheses thrombosis (SAVORY registry and RESOLVE registry), and find out that therapeutic anticoagulation with warfarin, but not therapy with antiplatelet drugs, prevented and effectively treated this phenomenon. Better characterization of this observation is needed to determine its frequency and evaluate its clinical effect [50].

Durability: intermediate surgical-risk patients are expected to survive longer after TAVI when compared to higher-risk patients; the broad application of TAVI in low-risk patients should be limited until in vivo durability results are available for the TAVI prostheses [48]. While structural valve deterioration in surgically replaced valves has been thoroughly investigated, long-term follow-up data for TAVI valves implanted in patients remain sparse [48].

8. Conclusions

Nowadays, the patients with intermediate risk are in the frontier of TAVI and surgical AVR, and more than ever, the heart team has to be more accurate to choose between the different treatment options available. Current expansion of TAVI into lower surgical risk patients encourages the need to remain cautious about unbridled expansion into those patients, as many questions remain about valve durability, leaflet thrombosis, and higher rates of paravalvular leak and permanent pacemakers [48]. Meanwhile, the surgical approach has improved and evolved to a reduction in surgical aggression. TAVI and minimally invasive aortic valve replacement [51] have become alternatives to surgical aortic valve replacement via median sternotomy (SAVR) to treat severe aortic stenosis (AS). Despite increased interest and utilization, few studies have directly compared TAVI and miniAVR. MiniAVR maintains potential advantages over SAVR, including the implantation of a durable prosthesis and low rates of perioperative myocardial infarction and paravalvular leak. It is associated with longer aortic crossclamp and cardiopulmonary bypass (CPB) times; however, the use of rapid deployment valves can circumvent this. Studies comparing TAVI and miniAVR demonstrate decreased postoperative mortality, valvular regurgitation, and incidence of stroke in the miniAVR cohorts [51].

From economic point of view, it is clear that for high-risk operable patients, TAVI is currently a more expensive therapy and probably a less effective alternative to surgical AVR, with an incremental cost-effectiveness ratio (ICER) that may be acceptable for high-income countries, but definitely not for the moderate- or low-income countries [52]. When use of TAVI is extended to include a larger number of moderate- to low-risk patients suitable for AVR, overall economic results become less favorable. When manufacturers reduce the exuberant cost of the valve and its accessories, TAVI may become the predominant therapy for patients with severe aortic stenosis. [52].

Finally, it is clear that both strategies will be the cornerstones in the modern AVR era, but the situations in which to apply each strategy have not yet been clearly delineated. More studies are needed to compare TAVI and miniAVR in low- and intermediate-risk patients. However, the current practice guidelines give a good pathway to choose the adequate therapeutic option in each individual case.

Acknowledgements

We want to give thanks to the cardiac surgery team at Policlinica de Guipuzcoa and Hospital Clinico Universitario de Valladolid, and especially to our colleagues: I. Gallo, A. Saenz, I. Perez-Moreiras, and A. Granda y E. Berruti.

Appendix

	Favor TAVI	Patient	Favor AVR	Patient
Clinical characteristic				
STS/EuroScore II < 4% (EuroScore I < 10%)			+	
STS/EuroScore II > 4% (EuroScore I > 10%)	+			
Severe comorbidities	+			
Age <75 years			+	
Age >75 years	+			
Previous cardiac surgery	+			
Frailty	+			
Restricted mobility	+			
Suspicion of Endocarditis			+	
Anatomical and technical aspects				
Favorable access for transfemoral TAVI	+			
Unfavorable access for TAVI			+	
Sequelae of chest radiation	+			
Porcelain aorta	+			
Pervious and permeable CABG	+			
Expected patient-prosthesis mismatch	+			
Severe chest deformation	+			
Short distance between coronary ostia and aortic valve annulus			+	
Aortic root morphology unfavorable for TAVI (Bicuspid valve, severe calcification)			+	
Undergoing CABG or another cardiac surgery			+	

Based on 2017 ESC/EACTS guidelines for the management of valvular heart disease [8].

Table A1.
Checklist for choice of therapeutic intervention option.

Author details

Omer Leal[1*], Diego Sanchez-Valenzuela[1] and Juan Bustamante-Munguira[2]

1 Department of Cardiovascular Surgery, Policlínica de Gipuzkoa, San Sebastian, Spain

2 Department of Cardiovascular Surgery, Hospital Clínico Universitario de Valladolid, Valladolid, Spain

*Address all correspondence to: omerleal82@gmail.com

References

[1] Schmitto JD, Mohr FW, Cohn LH. Minimally invasive aortic valve replacement: How does this perform in high-risk patients? Current Opinion in Cardiology. 2011;**26**(2):118-122

[2] Chambers JB. Aortic stenosis. European Journal of Echocardiography. 2009;**10**(1):i11-i19

[3] Freeman RV, Otto CM. Spectrum of calcific aortic valve disease: Pathogenesis, disease progression, and treatment strategies. Circulation. 2005;**111**(24):3316-3326

[4] Otto CM, Lind BK, Kitzman DW, Gersh BJ, Siscovick DS. Association of aortic-valve sclerosis with cardiovascular mortality and morbidity in the elderly. The New England Journal of Medicine. 1999;**341**(3):142-147

[5] Kurtz CE, Otto CM. Aortic stenosis: Clinical aspects of diagnosis and management, with 10 illustrative case reports from a 25-year experience. Medicine (Baltimore). 2010;**89**(6):349-379

[6] Ross J Jr, Braunwald E. Aortic stenosis. Circulation. 1968;**38**(1 Suppl):61-67

[7] Nishimura RA, Otto CM, Bonow RO, Carabello BA, Erwin JP III, Guyton RA, et al. 2014 AHA/ACC guideline for the management of patients with valvular heart disease: Executive summary: A report of the American College of Cardiology/American Heart Association task force on practice guidelines. Circulation. 2014;**129**:2440-2492

[8] Baumgartner H, Falk V, Bax JJ, De Bonis M, Hamm C, Holm PJ, et al. ESC/EACTS Guidelines for the management of valvular heart disease. European Heart Journal. 2017;**38**(36):2739-2791. DOI: 10.1093/eurheartj/ehx391

[9] Baumgartner H, Hung J, Bermejo J, Chambers JB, Edvardsen T, Goldstein S, et al. Focus update on the echocardiographic assessment of aortic valve stenosis: EAE/ASE recommendations for clinical practice. European Heart Journal Cardiovascular Imaging. 2017;**18**:254-275

[10] Rafique AM, Biner S, Ray I, Forrester JS, Tolstrup K, Siegel RJ. Metanalysis of prognostic value of stress testing in patients with asymptomatic severe aortic stenosis. The American Journal of Cardiology. 2009;**104**:972-977

[11] Marechaux S, Hachicha Z, Bellouin A, Dumesnil JG, Meimoun P, Pasquet A, et al. Usefulness of exercise-stress echocardiography for risk stratification of true asymptomatic patients with aortic valve stenosis. European Heart Journal. 2010;**31**:1390-1397

[12] Steadman CD, Ray S, Ng LL, McCann GP. Natriuretic peptides in common valvular heart disease. Journal of the American College of Cardiology. 2010;**55**:2034-2048

[13] Bergler-Klein J, Klaar U, Heger M, Rosenhek R, Mundigler G, Gabriel H, et al. Natriuretic peptides predict symptom-free survival and postoperative outcome in severe aortic stenosis. Circulation. 2004;**109**:2302-2308

[14] Monin JL, Lancellotti P, Monchi M, Lim P, Weiss E, Piérard L, et al. Risk score for predicting outcome in patients with asymptomatic aortic stenosis. Circulation. 2009;**120**:69-75

[15] Lancellotti P, Moonen M, Magne J, O'Connor K, Cosyns B, Attena E, et al. Prognostic effect of long-axis left ventricular dysfunction and B-type natriuretic peptide levels in asymptomatic aortic stenosis. The

American Journal of Cardiology. 2010;**105**:383-388

[16] Musa TA et al. Myocardial scar and mortality in severe aortic stenosis: Data from the BSCMR Valve Consortium. Circulation. 2018;**138**:1935. DOI: 10.1161/CIRCULATIONAHA.117.032839

[17] Leal O, Bustamante J, Cánovas S, Pinto A. New therapeutic approaches to conventional surgery for aortic stenosis in high-risk patients. In: Aikawa E, editor. Calcific Aortic Valve Disease. Rijeka, Croatia: IntechOpen; 2013. pp. 451-482. DOI: 10.5772/54333. ISBN: 978-953-51-1150-4

[18] Nishimura RA, Otto CM, Bonow RO, Carabello BA, Erwin JP 3rd, Fleisher LA, et al. 2017 AHA/ACC focused update of the 2014 AHA/ACC guideline for the management of patients with valvular heart disease: A report of the American College of Cardiology/American Heart Association task force on clinical practice guidelines. Circulation. 2017;**135**:e1159-e1195. DOI: 10.1161/CIR.0000000000000503

[19] Otto CM, Kumbhani DJ, Alexander KP, Calhoon JH, Desai MY, Kaul S, et al. 2017 ACC expert consensus decision pathway for transcatheter aortic valve replacement in the management of adults with aortic stenosis. Journal of the American College of Cardiology. 14 March 2017;**69**(10):1313-1346. DOI: 10.1016/j.jacc.2016.12.006

[20] Iung B, Laouénan C, Himbert D, et al. Predictive factors of early mortality after transcatheter aortic valve implantation: Individual risk assessment using a simple score. Heart. 2014;**100**:1016-1023

[21] Edwards FH, Cohen DJ, O'Brien SM, et al. Development and validation of a risk prediction model for in-hospital mortality after transcatheter aortic valve replacement. JAMA Cardiology. 2016;**1**(1):46-52. DOI: 10.1001/jamacardio.2015.0326

[22] Beckmann A, Hamm C, Figulla HR, Cremer J, Kuck KH, Lange R, et al. The German Aortic Valve Registry (GARY): A nationwide registry for patients undergoing invasive therapy for severe aortic valve stenosis. The Thoracic and Cardiovascular Surgeon. 2012;**60**:319-325. DOI: 10.1055/s-0032-1323155

[23] The STS/ACC TAVR In-Hospital Mortality Risk App [Internet]. 2018. Available from: https://www.acc.org/tools-and-practice-support/mobile-resources/features/tavr-in-hospital-mortality-risk-app

[24] Stortecky S, Schoenenberger AW, Moser A, Kalesan B, Juni P, Carrel T, et al. Evaluation of multidimensional geriatric assessment as a predictor of mortality and cardiovascular events after transcatheter aortic valve implantation. JACC. Cardiovascular Interventions. 2012;**5**:489-496

[25] Dimitri A et al. Agreement between the new EuroSCORE II, the Logistic EuroSCORE and the Society of Thoracic Surgeons score: Implications for transcatheter aortic valve implantation. Archives of Cardiovascular Diseases. 2014;**107**(6-7):353-360. DOI: 10.1016/j.acvd.2014.05.002

[26] Harken DE, Soroff HS, Taylor WH. Aortic valve replacement. In: Merendino KA, editor. Prosthetic Valves for Cardiac Surgery. Springfield, IL: Thomas; 1961. pp. 508-526

[27] Starr A, Edwards ML. Mitral replacement: Clinical experience with a ball-valve prosthesis. Annals of Surgery. 1961;**154**:726-740

[28] Wu Y, Jin R, Gao G, Grunkemeier GL, Starr A. Cost-effectiveness of aortic valve replacement in the elderly: An introductory study. The Journal of Thoracic and Cardiovascular Surgery. 2007;**133**(3):608-613

[29] Bonacchi M, Prifti E, Giunti G, Frati G, Sani G. Does ministernotomy improve postoperative outcome in aortic valve operation? A prospective randomized study. The Annals of Thoracic Surgery. 2002;**73**(2):460-465

[30] Candaele S, Herijgers P, Demeyere R, Flameng W, Evers G. Chest pain after partial upper versus complete sternotomy for aortic valve surgery. Acta Cardiologica. 2003;**58**(1):17-21

[31] Liu J, Sidiropoulos A, Konertz W. Minimally invasive aortic valve replacement (AVR) compared to standard AVR. European Journal of Cardio-Thoracic Surgery. 1999;**16** (Suppl 2):S80-S83

[32] Moustafa MA, Abdelsamad AA, Zakaria G, Omarah MM. Minimal vs median sternotomy for aortic valve replacement. Asian Cardiovascular & Thoracic Annals. 2007;**15**(6):472-475

[33] Bustamante J, Cánovas S, Fernández AL. Minimally invasive aortic valve surgery—New solutions to old problems. In: Hirota M, editor. Aortic Stenosis—Etiology, Pathophysiology and Treatment. Rijeka, Croatia: InTech; 2012. pp. 91-114. DOI: 10.5772/19831

[34] Grossi EA, Galloway AC, Ribakove GH, Zakow PK, Derivaux CC, Baumann FG, et al. Impact of minimally invasive valvular heart surgery: A case control study. The Annals of Thoracic Surgery. 2001;**71**(3):807-810

[35] Flameng W, Herregods MC, Hermans H, Van der Mieren G, Vercalsteren M, Poortmans G, et al. Effect of sutureless implantation of the Perceval S aortic valve bioprosthesis on intraoperative and early postoperative outcomes. The Journal of Thoracic and Cardiovascular Surgery. 2011;**142**(6):1453-1457

[36] Shrestha M, Folliguet T, Meuris B, Dibie A, Bara C, Herregods MC, et al. Sutureless Perceval S aortic valve replacement: A multicenter, prospective pilot trial. The Journal of Heart Valve Disease. 2009;**18**(6):698-702

[37] Shrestha M, Fischlein T, Meuris B, Flameng W, Carrel T, Madonna F, et al. European multicentre experience with the sutureless Perceval valve: Clinical and haemodynamic outcomes up to 5 years in over 700 patients. European Journal of Cardio-Thoracic Surgery. 2016;**49**:234-241

[38] Günther L, Dominik W. Chitwood Walter Randolph. Rapid-deployment valves: Finally the fog is lifting-benefits beyond crossclamp and bypass times. The Journal of Thoracic and Cardiovascular Surgery. 2017;**154**: 1527-1531. 10.1016/J. JTCVS.2017.06.065

[39] Borger MA, Moustafine V, Conradi L, Knosalla C, Richter M, Merk DR, et al. A randomized multicenter trial of minimally invasive rapid deployment versus conventional full sternotomy aortic valve replacement. The Annals of Thoracic Surgery. 2015;**99**:17-25

[40] Kocher AA, Laufer G, Haverich A, Shresta M, Walther T, Misfeld M, et al. One-year outcomes of the surgical treatment of aortic stenosis with a next generation surgical aortic valve (TRITON) trial: A prospective multicentre study of rapid-deployment aortic valve replacement with the EDWARDS INTUITY valve system. The Journal of Thoracic and Cardiovascular Surgery. 2013;**145**:110-116

[41] Barnhart GR, Accola KD, Grossi EA, Woo YJ, Mumtaz MA, Sabik JF, et al. TRANSFORM (Multicenter Experience With Rapid Deployment Edwards INTUITY Valve System for Aortic Valve Replacement) US clinical trial: Performance of a rapid deployment aortic valve. The Journal of Thoracic and Cardiovascular Surgery. 2017;**153**:241-51.e242

[42] Cribier A, Eltchaninoff H, Bash A, Borenstein N, Tron C, Bauer F, et al. Percutaneous transcatheter implantation of an aortic valve prosthesis for calcific aortic stenosis: First human case description. Circulation. 2002;**106**(24):3006-3008

[43] Holmes DR Jr, Mack MJ. Transcatheter valve therapy a professional society overview from the American college of cardiology foundation and the society of thoracic surgeons. Journal of the American College of Cardiology. 2011;**58**(4):445-455

[44] Mack MJ et al. 5-year outcomes of transcatheter aortic valve replacement or surgical aortic valve replacement for high surgical risk patients with aortic stenosis (PARTNER 1): A randomised controlled trial. Lancet. 2015;**385**:2477-2484. 10.1016/S0140-6736(15)60308-7

[45] Généreux P, Webb JG, Svensson LG, et al. Vascular complications after transcatheter aortic valve replacement: Insights from the PARTNER (Placement of AoRTic TraNscathetER valve) trial. Journal of the American College of Cardiology. 2012;**60**:1043-1052

[46] Martin B, Leon MB, et al. Transcatheter or surgical aortic-valve replacement in intermediate-risk patients. The New England Journal of Medicine. 2016;**374**:1609-1620. DOI: 10.1056/NEJMoa1514616

[47] Reardon MJ, Van Mieghem NM, Popma JJ, et al. Surgical or transcatheter aortic-valve replacement in intermediate-risk patients. The New England Journal of Medicine. 2017;**376**:1321-1331

[48] Arora S, Vavalle JP. Transcatheter aortic valve replacement in intermediate and low risk patients-clinical evidence. Annals of Cardiothoracic Surgery. 2017;**6**(5):493-497. DOI: 10.21037/acs.2017.07.01

[49] Escutia-Cuevas HH, Merino-Rajme JA, Alcántara-Meléndez MA, et al. TAVI in intermediate-risk patients: A review in purpose of a case. Revista Mexicana de Cardiología. 2018;**29**(2):102-111

[50] Makkar RR, Fontana G, Jilaihawi H, et al. Possible subclinical leaflet thrombosis in bioprosthetic aortic valves. The New England Journal of Medicine. 2015;**373**:2015-2024. DOI: 10.1056/NEJMoa1509233

[51] Hoffmann CT, Heiner JA, Nguyen TC. Review of minimal access versus transcatheter aortic valve replacement for patients with severe aortic stenosis. Annals of Cardiothoracic Surgery. 2017;**6**(5):498-503. DOI: 10.21037/acs.2017.09.02

[52] Manolis AS. Transcatheter aortic valve implantation economics: A grisly reality. Annals of Cardiothoracic Surgery. 2017;**6**(5):516-523. DOI: 10.21037/acs.2017.07.02

Chapter 4

Transcatheter Aortic Valve Replacement: Clinical Indications and Outcomes

Naresh Kumar Monigari and Anoop Agarwal

Abstract

Severe calcific aortic stenosis (AS) is commonly seen in the elderly population, and as human longevity increases, the prevalence of severe AS is bound to increase. Symptomatic severe AS, if left untreated, carries high mortality with 2-year survival below 50%. Surgical aortic valve replacement (SAVR) had been the standard of care for such patients with excellent outcome. As the patient's comorbidities increase, so does surgical risk for SAVR. Since its first human use in 2002 and commercial approval in 2007 (CE mark, Europe), transcatheter aortic valve replacement (TAVR) has come up as an excellent alternative to SAVR in patients with higher surgical risk profile. Iterations in device design added to enhanced operator experience can be attributed towards improved clinical outcomes. Indications for TAVR continues to expand and now includes patients with intermediate surgical risk as well. This chapter discusses indications and evidence for TAVR and touches upon patient selection and complications after TAVR.

Keywords: severe aortic stenosis, transcatheter aortic valve replacement, indications of TAVR, complications of TAVR, trials on TAVR

1. Introduction

A population-based study done by Eveborn et al. demonstrated an increase in the prevalence of AS with age, from 0.2% at 50–59 years to 9.8% at 80–89 years [1].

Prevalence of any AS and severe AS from pooled data involving multiple studies was shown to be 12.5 and 3.4% respectively among people of age >75. Approximately half to one-third of patients with severe AS may be asymptomatic at the time of diagnosis [2].

Due to long asymptomatic period associated with severe Aortic stenosis, patients may not report any overt symptoms, or compensate for their decreased exertional capacity by slowing down their daily activities attributing it to normal aging. Addressing symptom onset in patients with severe AS is extremely important as the onset of symptoms markedly decreases survival unless aortic valve replacement is performed.

Early observation done by Ross and Braunwald [3] showed that patients with angina have a 50% 5-year survival rate without AVR, those with syncope have 50% 3-year survival. Heart failure carries worse prognosis with mean survival rate of less than 2 years without AVR.

1) As a bridge to future definitive therapy: a) Hemodynamically unstable, b) Bridge to TAVR/SAVR in patients with reversible comorbidities, c) Need for percutaneous coronary intervention 2. As a palliative measure for symptomatic severe AS with poor life expectancy due to non-cardiac comorbidities who are considered poor candidates for TAVR/SAVR 3. Combined with TAVR, as in balloon expandable valves 4. Symptomatic patient before undergoing emergent non cardiac surgery 5. To assess contribution of AS for symptom status in presence of severe concomitant pulmonary involvement 6. Patients with congenital aortic stenosis 7. Symptomatic severe aortic stenosis in pregnant patients when optimal medical therapy fails.

Table 1.
Indications for balloon aortic valvuloplasty (BAV).

While SAVR is considered standard of care for management of symptomatic severe aortic stenosis, one-third of patients with severe AS with indications for SAVR may be denied surgery in view of advanced age and comorbidities.

Catheter-based balloon aortic valvuloplasty (BAV) was developed in 1985 as a less invasive solution for patients with symptomatic severe AS who were denied SAVR.

High rates of recurrence (80%) at 1 year associated with BAV hindered its widespread adaptability and search for other less invasive therapeutic option for severe AS patients was continued.

Contemporary indications for BAV are listed in **Table 1**. Currently, BAV is reserved for use as a bridge-to-decision to provide more definitive therapy for AS and for patients with contraindications for TAVR in whom relief of Aortic obstruction will improve quality of life.

2. TAVR: early concepts

To circumvent restenosis after BAV, a combination of stent frame and valve within was thought as an alternative. This arrangement could potentially implant an aortic valve in place of diseased native aortic valve using minimally invasive catheterization technique, thus avoiding high morbidity and mortality associated with high risk SAVR. Routine observation of high-pressure balloon inflation (4–5 atmospheres) leading to opening of all calcified aortic valves in a circular fashion led to the concept of TAVR [4].

In 1992, Andersen and colleagues [5], used a hand-made porcine valve contained within a metallic mesh and successfully implanted at various cardiac sites in a pig model. This was the first evidence of use of a stented valve.

In 1999 percutaneous valve technologies (PVT) designed early models of balloon expandable transcatheter heart valve (THV) [4].

The first human implantation of a percutaneous stented valve to a degenerated right ventricle-to-pulmonary artery conduit was done in 2000 by Bonhoeffer and colleagues [6]. This was a bovine jugular valve mounted on stent platform.

After initial success with the sheep model, Dr. Alain Cribier and his team performed the first successful TAVR in human using a balloon expandable THV on 16th April 2002 as a bailout procedure after failed emergency BAV [4].

3. Evolution of TAVR: indications and clinical trial evidence for TAVR

After initial success with the Sheep model, first human implantation with the balloon expandable Edwards valve was done on 16th April 2002 after failed emergency BAV as a bailout procedure [4].

After encouraging initial results, Dr. Cribier and team were able to recapitulate TAVR in a few patients. Worldwide demonstrations of this innovative therapy led to its increased acceptance. TAVR was transforming from a crazy idea to a viable therapy option. The Cribier valve technology was acquired by Edwards Lifesciences (Irvine, CA) for further development, and the THV was further marketed as Edwards Sapien valve.

Simultaneously scientists from Europe were working on a self-expandable valve (CoreValve, Medtronic, Inc.; Minneapolis, MN) platform as an alternative to balloon expandable valve since 2004 and human implantations were being done successfully.

As the number of TAVR implantations increased, data from multiple small studies and registries like SOURCE, ADVANCE, FRANCE I and FRANCE II showed procedural success (30 days survival) ranging from 67–92%.

With the available data, the European CE mark authorization was granted in August 2007 for the Edwards Sapien balloon expandable THV with the transfemoral RetroFlex delivery system and in January 2008 for use with the transapical Ascendra delivery device.

PARTNER was the first randomized trial that compared TAVR with standard therapy. Cohort B of this landmark trial demonstrated superiority of TAVR over medical therapy in patients with severe symptomatic AS who were considered extreme (or prohibitive) risk for SAVR. At 1 year follow up, absolute risk reduction in all-cause mortality of 20% was observed, a finding which held true even at 5 years follow up [7].

Cohort A of PARTNER trial compared TAVR with SAVR and showed that TAVR was non-inferior to SAVR in patients with high surgical risk (society of thoracic surgeons (STS) score >8%). CoreValve extreme risk trial data showed benefit of TAVR with reduction in all-cause mortality.

In November 2011, United States Food and Drug Administration (US FDA) approved TAVR as a treatment option for patients with symptomatic severe AS who were considered inoperable for SAVR. Favourable clinical data using self-expanding THV CoreValve (Medtronic) led to its USFDA approval in 2014 on similar patient subset.

With the available evidence from randomised control trials (RCTs) and multiple registry data, TAVR was given Class I LOE B recommendation in patients with prohibitive (not suitable for SAVR) and increased surgical risk by ESC guidelines [8] and Class I LOE A by ACC/AHA guidelines [9].

Another important observation noted in PARTNER 1 trial was diminishing survival benefit of TAVR with higher STS score. This led to stress more importance on patient selection.

Intermediate surgical risk (STS score ≥4–8%) patients with symptomatic severe AS were enrolled in PARTNER 2 trial comparing TAVR using second generation Sapien valve (Sapien XT) with SAVR along with subgroup analysis of transfemoral and transthoracic cohorts. All-cause mortality in TAVR arm was non-inferior to SAVR at 2 years with comparable stroke and permanent pacemaker rates.

The SURTAVI (surgical replacement and transcatheter aortic valve implantation) trial used Self-expandable CoreValve and enrolled patients with symptomatic severe AS with intermediate surgical risk and showed all-cause mortality in TAVR group non-inferior to SAVR at 1 and 2 years.

PARTNER 2 and SURTAVI trials also showed a favourable decreasing trend in all-cause mortality and post-procedure stroke rates (refer to **Table 2**).

ACC/AHA has given Class II LOE (level of evidence) A recommendation for TAVR in intermediate-risk population [9].

With the availability of 5-year data on TAVR showing good valve durability, focus of attention shifted to extend the benefit of TAVR to low-risk population with severe AS.

NOTION trial [10] and low-risk TAVR trial [11] evaluated the role of TAVR in low-risk population (STS score <4%).

NOTION trial is one of the earliest randomized trials, started recruiting patients in 2009 in a single centre. NOTION trial enrolled patients with symptomatic severe AS with low surgical risk and randomized them to TAVR versus SAVR. All-cause mortality at 1 year seen in this study was lower in TAVR arm compared to SAVR, an effect that persisted at 5 years.

The post-procedure permanent pacemaker implantation (PPI) rates and PVL (paravalvular leak) were higher in the TAVR group. Despite higher PPI and PVL rates, the all-cause mortality was lower with TAVR than SAVR. Higher PPI rates were because of an overenthusiastic approach for pacemaker implantation in view of lack of experience during those days.

The above-mentioned trials showed a consistent reduction in 30 days all-cause mortality attributed to improved technical advances, procedural skills and better patient selection (refer to **Table 2**).

SURTAVI 2012	PARTNER 2 2011	PARTNER B 2007	PARTNER A 2007	**Clinical Trial**
Severe AS with intermediate risk (STS ≥3 and ≤15)	Severe AS with intermediate risk (STS ≥4)	Severe AS with high risk and not suitable for SAVR. (Assessed by 2 CT surgeons and 1 Cardiologist)	Severe AS with high risk (STS PROM ≥10%)	**Population studied**
TAVR(879) vs SAVR(867) Core valve	TAVR (1011) vs SAVR(1021) Sapien XT valve	TAVR (179) vs Medical (179) 1st gen Edward Sapien	TAVR (348) vs SAVR (351) 1st gen Edward Sapien	**Comparator& valve used**
All-cause mortality TAVR vs. SAVR At 1 year 8.1% vs 8.8%	All-cause mortality TAVR vs. SAVR At 1 year 14.5% vs 16.4% At 2 year 19.3% vs 21.1%	All-cause mortality TAVR vs. medical therapy At 1 year 30.7% vs 50.7% At 2 years 43% vs 68% At 5 years 38.9% vs 66.7%	All-cause mortality TAVR vs. SAVR At 1 year 24.3% vs 26.8% At 2 year 33.9% vs 35%	**Primary end point**
At 1 year 8.2% vs 8.6% At 2 years 10% vs 11%	At 30 days 5.5% vs 6.1% At 1 year 10.1% vs 9.7%	At 1 year 11.2% vs 5.5% At 2 year 13.8% vs 5.5% At 5 year 16% vs 18.2%	At 1 yr. 8.7% vs 4.3% At 2 yrs. 11.2% vs 6.5%	**Stroke**
At 30 days 25.9% vs 6.6%	At 2 years 11.8% vs 10.3%	At 2 years 6.4% vs 8.6%	At 2 years 6.4% vs 7.2%	**Permanent pacemaker**
At 1 year 5.3% vs 0.8% At 2 years 5.8% vs 1.2%	Mod to severe PVL in At 1 yr. 3.4% vs. 0.4%	10% at 30 days had Moderate to severe PVL in TAVR	11.8% at 30 Days had Moderate to Severe PVL	**Paravalvular leak**

Core valve High risk 2011	Core valve extreme risk 2011	NOTION 2009	**Clinical Trial**
Severe AS determined as high risk by heart team (STS>15% and risk of death within 30days of surgery <50%)	Severe AS determined as high risk by heart team (STS>15% and risk of death within 30days of surgery >50%)	Severe AS, candidate suitable for TAVR and SAVR by multidisciplinary team	**Population studied**
TAVR (394) vs SAVR (401) Core valve	TAVR (506) Vs Prespecified Objective goal	TAVR (145) Vs SAVR (135) Core valve	**Comparator and** **Valve used**
All-cause mortality TAVR vs. SAVR At 1 year was 14.2% vs 19.1%	All-cause mortality at 1 year 8.4%TAVR vs. 24.3%OPG	All-cause mortality TAVR Vs. SAVR At 30 days 2.1% Vs. 3.7%. At 1 year 4.9% vs 7.5%	**Primary end point**
At 30 days 4.9% vs 6.2% At 1 year 8.8% vs 12.6%	Stroke was 4% at 30 days and 7% at 1 year	At 30 days 2.8% Vs 3% At 5 year 10.5% Vs 8.2%	**Stroke**
At 30 days 19.8% vs 7.1% At 1 year 22.3% vs 11.3%	At 30 days 21.6%	At 30 days 34.1% Vs 1.6%	**Permanent pacemaker**
At discharge 7.7% vs 0.3% At 1 year 6.1% vs 0.5%	10.7% at discharge and 4.3% at 1 year	15.7% Vs 0.9% at 1 year	**Paravalvular leak**

Table 2.
Clinical trials data.

A valve in valve (ViV), by virtue of the procedure being a re-do sternotomy, with patients typically in their 70 and 80s age, they usually fall into an intermediate risk category for surgical treatment. Most of the patients with degenerated bio prosthetic aortic valve qualify for TAVR.

The main issues with ViV are under expansion of the valve leading to higher gradients and a higher risk of coronary obstruction.

Bicuspid aortic valve (BiV), not approved, TAVR had been used off-label in BiV.

Issues related to the use of TAVR in BiV are:

Large annulus with severe and asymmetric calcification or presence of raphe can hinder with positioning and expansion of the valve that can lead to PVL or annulus rupture.

Increased risk of aortic dissection or rupture in view of concomitant aortopathy.

In view of relatively young patients with longer life expectancy, the durability of TAVR valve is still a concern.

A study by Ravi et al., which included 435 patients with BiV, showed higher 30 days all-cause mortality with off label TAVR (8.5%) when compared with on label TAVR (6.1%) [12].

Outcomes are not as favourable as tricuspid valve, still a valid alternative in patients with higher surgical risk profile.

4. Patient selection for TAVR

Patient evaluation is directed towards identifying patients where significant improvement in the quality and duration of life is expected with AVR and avoid unnecessary intervention where the benefit is unlikely due to other confounding co-morbidities.

Extreme comorbidities that overwhelm the benefit of TAVR may render the procedure futile as shown in PARTNER cohort B.

The essential components for patient selection include:

1. Clinical risk stratification with emphasis on heart team
2. Geriatric risk stratification
3. Anticipated clinical benefit and
4. Assessment of patient's goals and preferences
5. Anatomic assessment: MDCT as standard. 3D TEE as an alternative.
    a. Accurate valve sizing
    b. Vascular access planning

4.1 Clinical risk stratification

Important components of clinical risk stratification are mentioned in **Table 3**.

STS-PROM and Euroscore II are the two most commonly used integrated risk scoring calculators used to assess surgical risk.

STS risk scoring system had been extensively utilized in clinical decision making for TAVR. SAVR, components of which are showed in **Table 4**.

STS score <4% is low risk.

≥4%, <8% is intermediate risk.

>8% is high risk.

- **Age**
- **Number of comorbidities**
- **Severely reduced left ventricular function**
- **Low flow (low stroke volume index, <35 ml/m2)**
- **Severe myocardial fibrosis**
- **Severe concomitant mitral and/or tricuspid valve disease**
- **Severe pulmonary hypertension (PASP ≥60 mmHg)**
- **Severe lung disease, particularly oxygen dependent**
- **Advanced renal impairment (stages 4 and 5)**
- **Liver disease**
- **Very high STS score (predicted risk of mortality >15%)**

Table 3.
Clinical predictors of increased risk.

Age, gender, ethnicity Anaemia Renal function Sleep Apnoea Associated co-morbidities like DM, Lung disease Drug abuse Pneumonia Home Oxygen MI Heart Failure NYHA class Cardiogenic Shock Tachyarrhythmia's Bradyarrhythymias Steroids use previous cardiac arrest Number of Diseased Vessels Ejection Fraction Aortic Stenosis Valvular pathology in addition to AS	Prior CABG Peripheral artery disease COPD Frailty Porclein aorta Chest wall irradiation Chest wall deformity

Table 4.
Variables included in STS PROM and variables not included in STS PROM.

Concept of heart team: doctors from various specialties as a team need to evaluate TAVR patients.

Multidisciplinary team approach provides an opportunity for active participation of doctors from multiple specialties and share views on different aspects of patient health care and also to counsel patient relatives on an anticipated line of management.

The team should consist of referring physician, Clinical Cardiologist, Interventional cardiologist, cardiothoracic surgeon, Cardiac anaesthesiologist, dedicated cardiac imaging specialist, Valve clinic coordinator, dedicated nursing and catheterisation laboratory team.

4.2 Geriatric risk stratification

Beyond the traditional co-morbidities like DM and HTN, the elderly population also need particular attention in terms of advanced frailty, disability in activities of daily living, malnutrition, mobility impairment, low muscle mass and strength, cognitive impairment and mood disorders.

The commonly used assessment tools are shown in **Table 5**.

4.3 The anticipated benefit of TAVR

Trial evidence consistently shows, treatment with TAVR in patients with symptomatic severe AS results in reduction of all-cause mortality, improved duration of survival.

Patients symptomatic because of severe AS not because of other comorbidities have the greatest symptomatic benefit.

Patient pre-operative symptom status can be assessed by Kansas city cardiomyopathy questionnaire (KCCQ) [13] and can be followed up linearly.

• Frailty 5-meter gait speed Fried's frailty scale • Disability Activities of daily living (ADL) Instrumental activities of daily living (IADL) • Cognitive impairment Mini-Mental Status Examination (MMSE) • Mood disturbance Geriatric Depression Scale (GDS) • Malnutrition Albumin Mini-nutritional assessment • Charlson comorbidity index

Table 5.
Geriatric assessment tools.

4.4 Patients goals and preferences

The assessment of futility must include consideration of patient's values, goals, and preferences.

Shared decision-making requires both patient and provider share information, work toward a consensus and reach agreement on the course of action.

In the TAVR population, when benefit in symptom relief aligns with a patient's goals, care may not futile.

However, when life prolongation and symptom relief is not anticipated, care may be futile.

TAVR is not recommended in patients with a life expectancy of <1 year, or if the benefit of TAVR will be less obvious in the backdrop of multiple co-morbidities.

4.5 Anatomic assessment

Assessment of valve calcification, valve anatomy, annulus size, coronary height, an angle of implantation, size of sinuses of Valsalva, ascending aorta and peripheral vascular access by multidetector computerized tomography scan (MDCT) is an integral part of pre TVAR work up.

4.5.1 Aortic annulus

Annulus is a virtual ring formed by basal hinge points of the valve cusps. The measurement of annulus size is a very important step as it determines the size of the TAVR valve.

Prosthesis undersizing causes the risk of significant Paravalvular leak (PVL) or valve embolization, if oversized, disruption of the aortic root and cause annular rupture or impingement on conduction system and may cause bundle branch block or complete heart block.

Cardiac complications:	**TEE related**
Conduction abnormalities	Dental trauma
Tachyarrhythmia's	Oral bleeding
Paravalvular leak	Oesophangeal injury
Coronary obstruction	Oesophageal rupture
Valve embolization	
Valve thrombosis (clinical or subclinical)	
Cardiac tamponade	**Anaesthesia related**
Annular rupture	
Aortic dissection	
Non cardiac complications:	**Vascular**
Renal dysfunction	Dissection or perforation
Stroke	Retro-peritoneal hematoma
Major bleeding	Pseudo aneurysm
Acute kidney injury	
Access site related infection	

Table 6.
Complications of TAVR.

3D TEE and MDCT are the two most commonly used imaging methods for annulus measurement.

MDCT is a non-invasive procedure, the ability to measure annulus during any part of the cardiac cycle and provide additional information like valve calcification, distribution of valve calcification, sizes of sinus of valsalva (SOV), coronary ostia distance from the annulus, makes it imaging of choice unless contraindicated in view of kidney injury [14].

4.5.2 Vascular access planning

MDCT because of excellent resolution provides a virtual roadmap for vasculature and allows identification of vessel size, tortuosity, calcification, and luminal diameter, which allows the planning of access routes with a view to minimizing vascular complication rate.

5. Complications of TAVR

TAVR has seen an overall decline in peri-procedural complications over time, partly owing to newer technology and expertise.

Complications associated with TAVR are as listed in **Table 6**.

According to transcatheter valve therapy (TVT data), 30-day in-hospital mortality has decreased from 7.5% in 2012 to 4.6% in 2015 [15].

This part of the chapter briefly reviews about important complications post TAVR.

5.1 Major vascular access site complications

Access site complications incidence depends upon the method of localization and the location of the puncture site, the need for multiple punctures and the size of the sheath used. The incidence of major vascular complications showed a decreasing trend attributed to technical innovations reducing sheath size and valve delivery systems.

The overall major vascular complication rate was 17% in PARTNER 1 trial, decreased to 2.5% in low-risk TAVR trial [11], 2018 due to improvements in the sheath and valve delivery systems.

5.2 Permanent pacemaker implantation (PPI)

Need for PPI arises due to a complex interaction of the valve with the conduction system.

The incidence of PPI has not decreased as expected, compared with other complications. Changes in the valve design to prevent PVL and position of valve implantation contributed for PPI.

PPI incidence appears to increase with the oversizing of the valve and changes in valve design to prevent PVL. Shallow implantation and improvement in technical skill could decrease the incidence of PVL as shown in the REPRISE trial.

PPI frequency varies in relation to the valve type used. Balloon Expandable valve has a relatively less incidence of PPI at the cost of higher valvular gradients.

The incidence of new PPI post-TAVR was 6–10% in PARTNER 1 and PARTNER 2 trials which is similar to 5% seen in low-risk TAVR study [11].

The requirement of PPI has been associated with increased hospital stay and financial burden but has not been shown to increase mortality conclusively.

5.3 Paravalvular leak (PVL)

PVL occurs because of the difference in the shape of the valve which is circular compared to the elliptical aortic annulus.

The incidence of PVL is consistently shown to be higher with TAVR than SAVR in all landmark trials of TAVR.

Valve size, aortic valve distribution of calcium and implantation depth were predictive of post TAVR PVL [16].

Precise annulus sizing by appropriate aortic imaging pre-TAVR is fundamental to prevent PVL. With the use of newer imaging technology and understanding of the factors involved the incidence of moderate or severe PVL decreased 12.5% in PARTNER B to <1% in low-risk TAVR data [11]. Out of 12.5% moderate to severe PVL in PARTNER cohort B only 0.7% have severe leak, severe PVL causing an increase in mortality or need for re-intervention is very rare.

5.4 Stroke

Stroke is one of the most devastating complication post-TAVR, it causes an increase in mortality, significant worsening of quality of life and disability.

A stroke occurs due to the embolization of plaque contents from atheroma disrupted during delivery system manipulations. Early trial PARTNER 1 used a balloon-expandable valve with a 22-24F delivery catheter and showed a 30-day stroke risk of 5.5–6.2% [7].

The risk of stroke decreased over the years with increasing operator experience, advancements in valve technology, and improvement in patient selection.

PARTNER 2 and CoreValve studies used Sapien XT and CoreValve which used 18F delivery catheter and showed a 30-day risk of stroke around 4% [17–19].

A study on the timing of stroke post-TAVR by Samir et al. showed that of strokes occurring within 30 days post-TAVR, 64% were diagnosed within 2 days and 85% were diagnosed within 1 week, the risk of stroke after the initial peri-procedural period is not high [20]. More balloon post dilations and lack of dual antiplatelet therapy before the procedure were associated with a higher risk of early stroke [20].

Newer advances like Sentinel cerebral protection system are recently approved by the US FDA and are commercially available.

The Sentinel study investigated the role of Sentinel CPS (cerebral protection system) but failed to show a reduction in the median total new lesion volume on MRI. So In view of the lack of robust evidence regarding the efficacy of CPS, the choice of using neuroprotection in TAVR requires an individualized risk-benefit analysis.

Investigations therapies like protecting aortic arch vessels with CPS, excluding the LAA and refining post procedural antithrombotic strategy may aid in a further reduction in stroke incidence.

5.5 Durability

Structural valve deterioration is defined as any change in valve function resulting from an intrinsic abnormality leading to an intervention.

Increase in a mean gradient to >20 mm Hg or increase >10 mm Hg from baseline, an appearance of new valvular regurgitation constitutes SVD.

Rising interest for the use of TAVR in low-risk population makes durability of valve an important concern where the life expectancy of the patients would be more than 15 years. Five-year data from PARTNER 1 trial showed stable valve area and mean transvalvular gradient throughout the follow-up. The mean valve area was 1.52 cm^2 and the mean gradient was 10 mm Hg at 5 years and no events of clinical thrombosis of the TAVR valve [7].

Any increase in valvular gradients should warrant imaging workup for valve thrombosis. Data from multicentre registry showed, an incidence of VHD of 4.5% (overall VHD) and 2.8% within the first year (early VHD) [21].

Makkar et al. reported hypo-attenuated leaflet thickening (HALT) and reduced leaflet motion (RELM) in transcatheter valves, evaluated by four-dimensional volume-rendered computer tomography [22]. The effect of this finding on clinical outcomes needs further investigation.

Walksman et al. reported a 14% incidence of HALT and 11.2% RELM at 30 days post-TAVR, but were asymptomatic clinically.

Multivariate analysis showed the absence of anticoagulation at discharge, valve size <23 mm, a valve in valve procedure and greater BMI as predictors of transcatheter valve hemodynamic deterioration post-TAVR [21].

5.6 Miscellaneous

5.6.1 Annular rupture

Non-existent with self-expandable valves except in cases where pre or post-dilation is performed.

Because of the use of newer imaging modalities accurate sizing of the balloon, an annular rupture is a very rare phenomenon.

5.6.2 Valve embolization

Device embolization was defined as, Movement of valve prosthesis during or after deployment such that it loses contact with the aortic annulus. A study by Makkar et al., out of 2,554 patients who underwent TAVR, valve embolization was noted in 1% of patients. Technical factors like undersized valve and complex aortic valve anatomy, incomplete balloon inflation, and pacing failure were associated with valve embolization [23].

5.6.3 Coronary obstruction

Symptomatic coronary obstruction following TAVR is rare but a life-threatening complication. Multicentre registry data shows an incidence of 0.6%. It was observed more frequently with balloon expandable valve and in those with a previous surgical prosthesis [24]. Low lying coronary ostium and shallow sinus of Valsalva were anatomical factors associated with the risk for coronary obstruction [24].

5.6.4 Trans oesophageal echo (TEE) related complications

The incidence of complications with TEE is <1%. Dental trauma, oral bleeding, oesophageal erosions and rarely oesophageal rupture.

5.6.5 Anaesthesia-related complications

Respiratory dependence, hypotension, nausea and vomiting are among common, complete description of anaesthesia related complications is beyond the scope of this chapter.

6. Conclusion

TAVR, a novel approach started as an impossible idea, witnessed a remarkable journey and now is an established therapy in management of symptomatic severe Aortic stenosis patients. Outcomes post TAVR are bound to get better as technology improves and expertise increases. "TAVR first approach may be the future."

Acknowledgements

CARE Hospitals, Banjara Hills, Hyderabad.

Conflict of interest

There are no conflicts of interest.

Appendix

AS	aortic stenosis
STS PROM	society of thoracic surgeons, predicted risk of mortality
MI	myocardial infarction
V tach/V fib	ventricular tachycardia/ventricular fibrillation
CT surgeon	cardiothoracic surgeon
PPI	permanent pacemaker implantation
PVL	paravalvular leak
VARC	valve academic research consortium
CPS	cerebral protection system
LAA	left atrial appendage

VHD	valve hemodynamic deterioration
SVD	structural valve degeneration
TAVR	transcatheter aortic valve replacement
HALT	hypo attenuated leaflet thickening
RELM	reduced leaflet motion
COPD	chronic obstructive pulmonary disease
CABG	coronary artery bypass graft
BAV	balloon aortic valvuloplasty
THV	transcutaneous heart valve
PVT	percutaneous valve technologies
PARTNER	placement of aortic transcatheter valve trial
SOURCE	Sapien aortic bioprosthesis European Outcome Registry
NOTION	Nordic aortic valve intervention trial
SURTAVI	surgical replacement and transcatheter aortic valve implantation
SOV	sinus of valsalva
TVT	transcatheter valve therapy
TEE	trans oesophageal echo

Author details

Naresh Kumar Monigari* and Anoop Agarwal
CARE Hospitals, Hyderabad, India

*Address all correspondence to: medico.ktya@gmail.com

References

[1] Eveborn GW, Schirmer H, Heggelund G, Lunde P, Rasmussen K. The evolving epidemiology of valvular aortic stenosis the Tromso study. Heart (British Cardiac Society). 2013;**99**(6):396-400

[2] Osnabrugge RLJ, Mylotte D, Head SJ, Van Mieghem NM, Nkomo VT, LeReun CM, et al. Aortic stenosis in the elderly: Disease prevalence and number of candidates for transcatheter aortic valve replacement: A meta-analysis and modeling study. Journal of the American College of Cardiology. 2013;**62**(11):1002-1012

[3] Ross J Jr, Braunwald E. Aortic stenosis. Circulation. 1968;**38**(1 Suppl):61-67

[4] Cribier AG. The odyssey of TAVR from concept to clinical reality. Texas Heart Institute Journal. 2014;**41**(2):125-130

[5] Andersen HR, Knudsen LL, Hasenkam JM. Transluminal implantation of artificial heart valves. Description of a new expandable aortic valve and initial results with implantation by catheter technique in closed chest pigs. European Heart Journal. 1992;**13**(5):704-708

[6] Bonhoeffer P, Boudjemline Y, Saliba Z, Merckx J, Aggoun Y, Bonnet D, et al. Percutaneous replacement of pulmonary valve in a right-ventricle to pulmonary-artery prosthetic conduit with valve dysfunction. Lancet (London, England). 2000;**356**(9239):1403-1405

[7] Smith CR, Leon MB, Mack MJ, Miller DC, Moses JW, Svensson LG. et al., Transcatheter versus surgical aortic-valve replacement in high-risk patients. New England Journal of Medicine. 9 Jun 2011;**364**(23):2187-98. DOI: 10.1056/NEJMoa1103510

[8] Baumgartner H, Falk V, Bax JJ, De Bonis M, Hamm C, Holm PJ, et al. ESC/EACTS guidelines for the management of valvular heart disease. European Heart Journal. 2017;**38**(36):2739-2791

[9] Nishimura RA, Otto CM, Bonow RO, Carabello BA, Erwin JP, Fleisher LA, et al. 2017 AHA/ACC focused update of the 2014 AHA/ACC Guideline for the management of patients with valvular heart disease: A report of the American College of Cardiology/American Heart Association Task Force on Clinical Practice Guidelines. Circulation. 20 Jun 2017;**135**(25):e1159-e1195. DOI: 10.1161/CIR.0000000000000503

[10] Sondergaard L, Steinbruchel DA, Ihlemann N, Nissen H, Kjeldsen BJ, Petursson P, et al. Two-year outcomes in patients with severe aortic valve stenosis randomized to transcatheter versus surgical aortic valve replacement: The all-comers Nordic aortic valve intervention randomized clinical trial. Circulation. Cardiovascular Interventions. Jun 2016;**9**:(6). pii: e003665. DOI:10.1161/CIRCINTERVENTIONS.115.003665

[11] Waksman R, Rogers T, Torguson R, Gordon P, Ehsan A, Wilson SR, et al. Transcatheter aortic valve replacement in low-risk patients with symptomatic severe aortic stenosis. Journal of the American College of Cardiology. 2018;**72**(18):2095-2105

[12] Hira RS, Vemulapalli S, Li Z, McCabe JM, Rumsfeld JS, Kapadia SR, et al. Trends and outcomes of off-label use of transcatheter aortic valve replacement: Insights from the NCDR STS/ACC TVT registry. JAMA Cardiology. 2017;**2**(8):846-854

[13] Faller H, Steinbuchel T, Schowalter M, Spertus JA, Stork S, Angermann CE. The Kansas City cardiomyopathy questionnaire (KCCQ)—A new disease-specific quality of life measure for patients with chronic heart failure. Psychotherapie, Psychosomatik, Medizinische Psychologie. 2005;**55**(3-4):200-208

[14] Otto CM, Kumbhani DJ, Alexander KP, Calhoon JH, Desai MY, Kaul S, et al. 2017 ACC expert consensus decision pathway for transcatheter aortic valve replacement in the management of adults with aortic stenosis: A report of the American College of Cardiology Task Force on clinical expert consensus documents. Journal of the American College of Cardiology. 2017;**69**(10):1313-1346

[15] Grover FL, Vemulapalli S, Carroll JD, Edwards FH, Mack MJ, Thourani VH, et al. 2016 Annual Report of The Society of Thoracic Surgeons/American College of Cardiology Transcatheter Valve Therapy Registry. Journal of the American College of Cardiology. 2017;**69**(10):1215-1230

[16] Athappan G, Patvardhan E, Tuzcu EM, Svensson LG, Lemos PA, Fraccaro C, et al. Incidence, predictors, and outcomes of aortic regurgitation after transcatheter aortic valve replacement: Meta-analysis and systematic review of literature. Journal of the American College of Cardiology. 2013;**61**(15):1585-1595

[17] Leon MB, Smith CR, Mack MJ, Makkar RR, Svensson LG, Kodali SK, et al. Transcatheter or surgical aortic-valve replacement in intermediate-risk patients. New England Journal of Medicine. 28 Apr 2016;**374**(17):1609-20. DOI: 10.1056/NEJMoa1514616

[18] Popma JJ, Adams DH, Reardon MJ, Yakubov SJ, Kleiman NS, Heimansohn D, et al. Transcatheter aortic valve replacement using a self-expanding bioprosthesis in patients with severe aortic stenosis at extreme risk for surgery. Journal of the American College of Cardiology. 2014;**63**(19):1972-1981

[19] Adams DH, Popma JJ, Reardon MJ, Yakubov SJ, Coselli JS, Deeb GM, et al. Transcatheter aortic-valve replacement with a self-expanding prosthesis. The New England Journal of Medicine. 2014;**370**(19):1790-1798

[20] Kapadia S, Agarwal S, Miller DC, Webb JG, Mack M, Ellis S, et al. Insights into timing, risk factors, and outcomes of stroke and transient ischemic attack after transcatheter aortic valve replacement in the PARTNER trial (placement of aortic transcatheter valves). Circulation. Cardiovascular Interventions. Sep 2016;**9**(9). pii: e002981. DOI:10.1161/CIRCINTERVENTIONS.115.002981

[21] Del Trigo M, Munoz-Garcia AJ, Wijeysundera HC, Nombela-Franco L, Cheema AN, Gutierrez E, et al. Incidence, timing, and predictors of valve hemodynamic deterioration after transcatheter aortic valve replacement: Multicenter registry. Journal of the American College of Cardiology. 2016;**67**(6):644-655

[22] Makkar RR, Fontana G, Jilaihawi H, Chakravarty T, Kofoed KF, De Backer O, et al. Possible subclinical leaflet thrombosis in bioprosthetic aortic valves. The New England Journal of Medicine. 2015;**373**(21):2015-2024

[23] Makkar RR, Jilaihawi H, Chakravarty T, Fontana GP, Kapadia S, Babaliaros V, et al. Determinants and outcomes of acute transcatheter valve-in-valve therapy or embolization: A study of multiple valve implants in the U.S. PARTNER trial (placement

of AoRTic TraNscathetER valve trial Edwards SAPIEN transcatheter heart valve). Journal of the American College of Cardiology. 2013;**62**(5):418-430

[24] Ribeiro HB, Webb JG, Makkar RR, Cohen MG, Kapadia SR, Kodali S, et al. Predictive factors, management, and clinical outcomes of coronary obstruction following transcatheter aortic valve implantation: Insights from a large multicenter registry. Journal of the American College of Cardiology. 2013;**62**(17):1552-1562

Chapter 5

Infective Endocarditis in Aortic Valve Disease

Juan Bustamante-Munguira, Eva María Aguilar Blanco and Angels Figuerola-Tejerina

Abstract

Although infective endocarditis is a rare disease, its incidence has increased over the last years and, despite improved diagnosis and treatment, it has a poor prognosis. The left side is compromised in most cases and underlying valvular heart disease is present in a substantial proportion of cases. We review the incidence, main clinical features and indications for surgery in left-sided native valve infective endocarditis, focusing on the aortic valve.

Keywords: epidemiology, incidence, left-sided endocarditis, surgery

1. Introduction

Infective endocarditis (IE) is an infectious disease generally caused by bacteria that affect the endocardium, mostly the left chambers. Right-sided endocarditis is a different, much less prevalent entity with other clinical and epidemiological characteristics. In this chapter, we analyse left-sided endocarditis, focusing on aortic valve involvement to ascertain frequency of presentation, normal signs and symptoms, treatment and prognosis. Endocarditis frequently develops on a pathological valve. In the western world, the most common valve involvement is aortic sclerosis, that is, a certain degree of stenosis from age-associated valve degeneration. It is important to point out that aortic stenosis is the most prevalent western-world valvular heart disease that requires surgical or interventionist treatment. At 65 years of age, 2–7% of the population present some degree of aortic valve sclerosis, and the condition progresses over time [1–5].

Infective endocarditis is diagnosed based on modified Duke criteria. Their application means that there is an overlap with previously established criteria in large series. In addition, the European Society of Cardiology (ESC) in their Clinical Practice Guides have recently included some changes with respect to the criteria [6, 7], giving more importance to echocardiographic findings and the role of blood cultures. These findings are supported by new radiological tests, mainly CT scan, F-FDG PET/CT and radiolabelled leucocyte single-photon emission CT (SPECT)/CT, and there are a major criteria.

The incidence of IE is known to vary according to the series analysed. This finding might be due to multiple factors. Various epidemiological cohort studies covering prolonged time periods have recently been published, providing key updates to clinical and epidemiological knowledge about IE. What is observed in these series is an increase in IE incidence, greater comorbidity in the patients and a morbidity-mortality prognosis that has remained substantially the same during the last decades in spite of advances in diagnosis and therapy [8].

2. Incidence

As indicated earlier, infective endocarditis (IE) is a rare disease of poor prognosis, whose incidence has been growing during the last two decades. Various clinical pictures are found within it; fundamentally, it can be divided into endocarditis on native valve or prosthesis, and right- or left-sided endocarditis according to location [1–5]. Another entity has recently appeared that, due to its frequency and severity, is considered separate: health care-associated endocarditis.

Data on the incidence of the disease have been updated in the last few years by the publication of various studies of an epidemiological nature. The most recent ones report an incidence of 3–10 cases per 100,000 inhabitants/year, but there is great geographical variability in the data [1–5, 9]. Over the last few years, several groups have published incidences from local studies that give us a geographical view of the current IE situation. In a study carried out in Spain, Olmos et al. observed an increase in incidence, rising from 2.72 cases to 3.49 cases per 100,000 inhabitants/year during the period analysed (2003–2014) [10]. Likewise, Bustamante Munguira et al. reported increased IE incidence in Spain, which rose from 3.17% in 1997 to 5.56% in 2014 [9]. In Denmark, Erichsen et al. also observed a rise in incidence during 1994–2011, going from 3.93 to 7.55 cases per 100,000 inhabitants a year [11]. In Italy, Cresti et al. found 4.6 cases per 100,000 during the study period 1998–2014 [12]. Representing the Spanish Group Collaboration on Endocarditis (*Grupo de Apoyo al Manejo de Infective Endocarditis en España, GAMES*), Muñoz et al. estimated an annual incidence of 3.5 cases per 100,000 inhabitants during 2008–2012 [13].

The increase in the incidence of the disease is consequently perfectly documented in the different studies mentioned. One of the motives justifying this increase is the appearance of clinical practice-associated endocarditis, as we have pointed out. This type of endocarditis is becoming more and more frequent, reaching up to 25% depending on the series analysed. Other causes of increased IE incidence are population ageing and growth in patient comorbidity. As we indicated earlier, associated with ageing of the population, there is an increase in the prevalence of valvular heart disease, predominantly in the development of degenerative aortic sclerosis and degenerative mitral insufficiency.

Published records from different European countries reveal both increased IE incidence and increased fragility and comorbidity in patients presenting IE. In a study in France, Hoen et al. reported an incidence of 3.1 cases per 100,000 inhabitants a year [14]. In their study on an English population, Dayer et al. analysed the impact that the change in antibiotic prophylaxis recommendations had on the incidence of endocarditis in the United Kingdom. Their study results showed that IE incidence increased from the start of the study in 2000 until its end in 2013. The authors attributed this growth in incidence (as other authors have) to ageing of the population, increased comorbidity and the rise in invasive measures associated with health care attention. However, they also indicated that one of the determining factors in the sample analysed was the change in antibiotic prophylaxis recommendations instituted in March 2008 [15]. In the series reported by Erichsen et al., analysing the population in Denmark, incidence rose throughout the study period, from 3.93 per 100,000 inhabitants a year in 1994–1996 to 7.55 per 100,000 inhabitants a year in 2009–2011 **Table 1**.

Author	Country	Study period	No. of patients	Incidence	Rate of indication for surgery	Reference
Bustamante Munguira	Spain	1997–2014	34,399	3.17% in 1997 and 5.56% in 2014	11.7% in 1997 to 17.8% in 2014	[8]
Erichsen	Denmark	1994–2011	5486	3.93 in 1994–1996 to 7.55 in 2009–2011	None	[10]
Olmos	Spain	2003–2014	16,867	2.72 in 2003 3.49 in 2014	23%	[9]
Fedeli	Italy	2000–2008	1873	4.1 in 2000–2002 to 4.9 in 2006–2008	23%	[15]
Cresti	Italy	1998–2014	167	4.6/100,000	46.5%	[11]
Hoen	France	1999	390	3/100000	49%	[13]
Dayer	England	1 January 2004 to 31 March 2013	19,804	0.11 cases per 10 million people per month	None	[14]
Muñoz	Spain	1 January 2008 to 31 December 2012	1804	3.5 cases per 100,000 inhabitants	44.2%	[12]
Ilhão Moreira	Portugal	2006 and 2014	233		36.9%	[20]

Table 1.
Main epidemiological studies on endocarditis.

These epidemiological studies obtain the information from data in administrative databases gathered when patients are admitted. They are administrative coding systems used for management of both public and private hospitals. This method makes it possible to analyse broad population samples over long period of time, but the fact that it lacks clinical content is a decided weakness. This is the case with the Spanish series, in which the minimum basic data set of the National Surveillance System for Hospital Data in Spain provided by the Spanish Ministry of Health was used [9]. In Italy, Cresti et al. used the Health Care System Hospital Discharge Records database with a primary or secondary International Classification of Diseases 9th Revision IE diagnosis code [12]. The Danish registry published by Reichsen et al. was based on an analysis of the Danish National Patients Registry, which was set up in 1968 [11].

The data published in these studies should be interpreted with certain caution, given the limitations such analyses have. What is clear, and agreed upon in most of the studies, is that the incidence of endocarditis on both native and prosthetic valves has increased.

3. Left-sided endocarditis, with aortic compromise

When we analyse valve involvement, we see that endocarditis is found on left cavities in 90–95% of the cases, while right-side involvement is rare. Native valve endocarditis is far more common (70–80% of the cases) than prosthetic endocarditis [16]. Multiple valve involvement is infrequent, ranging up to 15–20% of the cases according to the series consulted [17].

According to the majority of authors, the frequency of distribution of mitral and aortic valve compromise follows a similar proportion. There are almost no studies that analyse aortic involvement individually [18]. This is not the case with native mitral valve endocarditis; some authors have analysed it independently, alleging that the embolism rate is greater and that surgical treatment for these patients can be based on valve repair with good short-, medium- and long-term clinical results. However, the majority of the studies do not discriminate according to location, making a global analysis. Nevertheless, there are certain discrepancies in the studies published.

In one of the most numerous series published, with 2781 patients attended in 58 centres from 25 countries, Murdoch et al. observed that the mitral valve was compromised in 41.1% of the cases, while the aortic valve was in 37.6% [19]. In a series of 945 consecutive episodes, Olmos et al. found no statistically significant differences between the two locations [20], while Muñoz et al. observed that the mitral valve was involved in 44.8% of the cases and the aortic in 47.2% [13].

There are discrepancies in the literature. In a French study with 303 patients with left-sided endocarditis, Lung et al. found a higher incidence of mitral valve compromise than of aortic (49.2 vs. 32.3%) [17]. At the opposite extreme, we find the results of the study by Ilhão Moreira et al.; in a series of 233 patients followed for 8 years, they observed that aortic involvement was more frequent (55.7%) than mitral (38.2%) [21].

As we have pointed out, it is important to remember that endocarditis develops on pathological valves in one-fourth of the cases, with valve degeneration being the most frequent underlying condition [10, 13, 19]. In some series, this percentage is even higher than 35% [12]. It bears repeating that epidemiological aspects are important in interpreting study results.

4. Specific clinical profile of left-sided infective endocarditis with aortic valve compromise

Independently of valve involvement, IE presents a shared clinical picture characterised by symptoms of systemic infection. Some of these are more frequent based on the location involved. The most common symptom is fever, which can be present in 90% of the patients. Heart failure is also highly frequent. Associated constitutional symptoms, such as weight loss, asthenia and anorexia, are also found. There are differences in the percentage of presentation in some of the complications.

4.1 Embolism

Aortic valve compromise does not involve embolic risk greater than that of the compromise of other valves. Its incidence depends on the size of the vegetation and of the microorganism causing the infection. The frequency of embolism in aortic endocarditis is, if anything, less than that of mitral endocarditis. Systemic embolism is estimated to occur in 22–50% of the cases; most embolisms affect the central nervous system, while other locations such as the spleen or kidney are less common [7, 22].

There is a certain variability in the results reported by different authors. Vilacosta et al., in a series of 211 patients with left-sided endocarditis, found a correlation between vegetation size and embolism for the patients with mitral valve endocarditis but not in the case of the aortic valve [23]. However, Hubert et al., in their study analysing 1022 patients, found no correlation with location, but did find a statistically significant association with vegetation size [24]. Likewise, in their study including 1456 patients, Rizzi et al. found no association with location but did find ones with vegetation size and with the causal agent being *S. aureus* [25].

When the relationship between microorganism and embolism is analysed, it can be observed that the results reported are also different according to the series considered. Vilacosta et al. indicated that they did not observe any differences based on the type of microorganism. This aspect is controversial, given that clinical practice guidelines and some authors point out that there is a relationship between endocarditis caused by specific microorganisms and the likelihood of developing embolic phenomena.

Various risk scores have been developed in relation to this complication for calculating the probability of developing embolisms. Among these, the Italian and French scales are the most utilised. In a study on 167 patients, Cresti et al. did not observe any differences between aortic and mitral locations in the case of native valve endocarditis [12]. Hubert et al., in a sample of 1022 patients, likewise found no relationship with location; however, they did observe an association with vegetation size and when the endocarditis was caused by *S. aureus* [24].

4.2 Atrioventricular block

Aortic valve compromise can progress with symptoms of aortic insufficiency. It may trigger heart failure if inception is acute, while other common symptoms are embolism and rhythm disorders. Within rhythm alterations, the most frequent complication is atrioventricular block from conduction system disruption; its incidence ranges from 1 to 15% depending on the series. This complication worsens the prognosis, principally because it is the consequence of an annular compromise reflecting the extension of the infection. It is more frequent when staphylococci are involved. In these cases, it is important to delay the pacemaker implantation and always be sure that the infectious process is under control, in order to avoid the risk of infection of the pacemaker. There are also differences in the literature as to the involvement of the aortic valve compared with the mitral, although some authors report similar figures [26].

4.3 Heart failure

Heart failure is the most frequent complication of patients with IE. It is the main factor that predicts mortality at 30 days [18]. The presence of heart failure is more common when the valve compromise is aortic. The mechanism that explains its appearance is the occurrence of valve dysfunction. It is currently the most common cause for indicating surgery [27, 28].

5. Indication for surgery in left-sided aortic valve endocarditis

The reported rate for indication for surgery also varies considerably according to the studies published. Surgery indication is influenced by the characteristics of the centre, which are basically determined by the availability of multidisciplinary teams in patient assessment. The range is very wide, going from very low figures of 9.6% of the patients with endocarditis [12] up to the rates of indication reported by Lung et al. of 73% of the patients attended (with surgery being performed in 46% of the cases) [17]. Analysed by location, aortic endocarditis required surgery in 38.2% of the cases, when aortic valve compromise was 17% lower.

Very few authors study surgery of the aortic valve independently of that of the mitral valve. The majority of the series combine the two in their analyses, considering them the same process, left-sided endocarditis. It should be remembered that there are some differences between the two locations with respect to clinical repercussion, the possibility of generating embolism and the appearance of rhythm disorders.

Bustamante Munguira et al., analysing the Spanish series during the time period 1997–2014, found that the percentage of patients requiring surgery increased over the course of the study, reaching 15.7% of the patients [9]. These figures are much lower than those of the European registry, in which the Euro Heart Survey reported a rate of 58.7% [29]. Once again, the most logical explanation for this finding lies in the establishment of protocols for and in the treatment of endocarditis with the attention of these patients being given by units of reference.

There are intermediate ranges between these figures. One example is the study by Murdoch et al. (with 2781 patients attended in 58 centres in 25 countries), in which 48.2% of the patients underwent surgery [19]. In this study, important differences based on the type of centre were also observed in the percentage of patients that received an indication for surgery, with ranges of 63.4–37.1% ($P < 0.001$). In the series reported by Olmos et al., 23% of the patients required surgery [10]; the percentage was greater in the case of the centres with cardiac surgery (35.5%). A limitation of this study was that it did not analyse the percentage of aortic patients compared with other patients having problems in different locations.

In the study published by Moreira et al. (analysing 233 patients for 8 years), 57% of the patients received the indication for surgery, and the patients were operated in 36.9% of the cases. In that study, the frequency of indication for surgical treatment was analysed according to location. It was found that operations were performed in 64% of the cases of aortic endocarditis, while the percentage was only 31% in the cases of mitral endocarditis [21].

6. Conclusions

Infective endocarditis has increased its frequency of appearance as a consequence of ageing of the population and of the number of invasive procedures giving rise to the appearance of the condition called health care-associated endocarditis. Left-sided cavities are compromised far more frequently than right-sided ones. However, there is no clear difference between the percentage of aortic and mitral valve involvement. Indications for surgery have gradually increased, but the result considered in terms of morbidity-mortality has not improved despite advances in techniques and postoperative care. It is hard to find studies in which aortic valve compromise is analysed individually, because most studies focus on studying left-cavity endocarditis and consequently produce a global evaluation.

Conflict of interest

None declared.

Author details

Juan Bustamante-Munguira[1]*, Eva María Aguilar Blanco[2] and
Angels Figuerola-Tejerina[3]

1 Department of Cardiac Surgery, Hospital Clinico Universitario de Valladolid, Valladolid, Spain

2 Department of Cardiac Surgery, Hospital Universitario 12 de Octubre, Madrid, Spain

3 Department of Prevention and Control of Infection, Hospital Universitario de La Princesa, Madrid, Spain

*Address all correspondence to: jbustamantemunguira@gmail.com

References

[1] Bor DH, Woolhandler S, Nardin R, Brusch J, Himmelstein DU. Infective endocarditis in the U.S., 1998-2009: A nationwide study. PLoS One. 2013;**8**:e60033

[2] Slipczuk L, Codolosa JN, Davila CD, Romero-Corral A, Yun J, Pressman GS, et al. Infective endocarditis epidemiology over five decades: A systematic review. PLoS One. 2013;**8**:e82665

[3] Pant S, Patel NJ, Deshmukh A, Golwala H, Patel N, Badheka A, et al. Trends in infective endocarditis incidence, microbiology, and valve replacement in the United States from 2000 to 2011. Journal of the American College of Cardiology. 2015;**65**:2070-2076

[4] Fedeli U, Schievano E, Buonfrate D, Pellizzer G, Spolaore P. Increasing incidence and mortality of infective endocarditis: A population-based study through a record-linkage system. BMC Infectious Diseases. 2011;**11**:48

[5] Aortic Stenosis. In: Hirota M, editor. Minimally Invasive Aortic Valve Surgery: New Solutions to Old Problems. Bustamante. ISBN 978-953-308-86-0

[6] Durack DT, Lukes AS, Bright DK. New criteria for diagnosis of infective endocarditis: Utilization of specific echocardiographic findings. Duke Endocarditis Service. The American Journal of Medicine. 1994;**96**:200-209

[7] Habib G, Lancellotti P, Antunes MJ, Bongiorni MG, Casalta JP, Del Zotti F, et al. 2015 ESC Guidelines for the management of infective endocarditis: The Task Force for the Management of Infective Endocarditis of the European Society of Cardiology (ESC). Endorsed by: European Association for Cardio-Thoracic Surgery (EACTS), the European Association of Nuclear Medicine (EANM). European Heart Journal. 2015;**36**(44):3075-3128

[8] Gelsomino S, Maessen JG, van der Veen F, Livi U, Renzulli A, Lucà F, et al. Emergency surgery for native mitral valve endocarditis: The impact of septic and cardiogenic shock. The Annals of Thoracic Surgery. 2012;**93**(5):1469-1476

[9] Bustamante-Munguira J, Mestres CA, Alvarez P, Figuerola-Tejerina A, Eiros Bachiller R, Gómez-Sánchez E, et al. Surgery for acute infective endocarditis: Epidemiological data from a Spanish nationwide hospital-based registry. Interactive Cardiovascular and Thoracic Surgery. 2018;**27**(4):498-504

[10] Olmos C, Vilacosta I, Fernández-Pérez C, Bernal JL, Ferrera C, García-Arribas D, et al. The evolving nature of infective endocarditis in Spain: A Population-Based Study (2003 to 2014). Journal of the American College of Cardiology. 2017;**70**(22):2795-2804

[11] Erichsen P, Gislason GH, Bruun NE. The increasing incidence of infective endocarditis in Denmark, 1994-2011. European Journal of Internal Medicine. 2016;**35**:95-99

[12] Cresti A, Chiavarelli M, Scalese M, Nencioni C, Valentini S, Guerrini F, et al. Epidemiological and mortality trends in infective endocarditis, a 17-year population-based prospective study. Cardiovascular Diagnosis and Therapy. 2017;**7**(1):27-35

[13] Muñoz P, Kestler M, De Alarcon A, Miro JM, Bermejo J, Rodríguez-Abella H, et al. Spanish Collaboration on Endocarditis-Grupo de Apoyo al Manejo de la Endocarditis Infecciosa en España (GAMES). Current Epidemiology and Outcome of Infective Endocarditis:

A Multicenter, Prospective, Cohort Study. Medicine (Baltimore). 2015;**94**(43):e1816

[14] Hoen B, Alla F, Selton-Suty C, Béguinot I, Bouvet A, Briançon S, et al. Association pour l'Etude et la Prévention de l'Endocardite Infectieuse (AEPEI) Study Group. Changing profile of infective endocarditis: Results of a 1-year survey in France. Journal of the American Medical Association. 2002;**288**(1):75-81

[15] Dayer MJ, Jones S, Prendergast B, Baddour LM, Lockhart PB, Thornhill MH. Incidence of infective endocarditis in England, 2000-13: A secular trend, interrupted time-series analysis. Lancet. 2015;**385**(9974):1219-1228

[16] López J, Revilla A, Vilacosta I, Sevilla T, García H, Gómez I, et al. Multiple-valve infective endocarditis: Clinical, microbiologic, echocardiographic, and prognostic profile. Medicine (Baltimore). 2011;**90**(4):231-236

[17] Iung B, Doco-Lecompte T, Chocron S, Strady C, Delahaye F, Le Moing V, et al. Cardiac surgery during the acute phase of infective endocarditis: Discrepancies between European Society of Cardiology guidelines and practices. European Heart Journal. 2016;**37**(10):840-848

[18] Mistiaen WP. What are the main predictors of in-hospital mortality in patients with infective endocarditis: A review. Scandinavian Cardiovascular Journal. 2018;**52**(2):58-68

[19] Murdoch DR, Corey GR, Hoen B, Miró JM, Fowler VG Jr, Bayer AS, et al. Clinical presentation, etiology, and outcome of infective endocarditis in the 21st century: The International Collaboration on Endocarditis-Prospective Cohort Study. Archives of Internal Medicine. 2009;**169**(5):463-473

[20] Olmos C, Vilacosta I, Fernández C, Sarriá C, López J, Del Trigo M, et al. Comparison of clinical features of left-sided infective endocarditis involving previously normal versus previously abnormal valves. The American Journal of Cardiology. 2014;**114**(2):278-283

[21] Ilhão Moreira R, Coutinho Cruz M, Moura Branco L, Galrinho A, Coutinho Miranda L, Fragata J, et al. Infective endocarditis: Surgical management and prognostic predictors. Revista Portuguesa de Cardiologia. 2018;**37**(5):387-394

[22] Bayer AS, Bolger AF, Taubert KA, et al. Diagnosis and management of infective endocarditis and its complications. Circulation. 1998;**98**:2936-2948

[23] Vilacosta I, Graupner C, San Román JA, Sarriá C, Ronderos R, Fernández C, et al. Risk of embolization after institution of antibiotic therapy for infective endocarditis. Journal of the American College of Cardiology. 2002;**39**(9):1489-1495

[24] Hubert S, Thuny F, Resseguier N, Giorgi R, Tribouilloy C, Le Dolley Y, et al. Prediction of symptomatic embolism in infective endocarditis: Construction and validation of a risk calculator in a multicenter cohort. Journal of the American College of Cardiology. 2013;**62**(15):1384-1392

[25] Rizzi M, Ravasio V, Carobbio A, Mattucci I, Crapis M, Stellini R, et al. Predicting the occurrence of embolic events: An analysis of 1456 episodes of infective endocarditis from the Italian Study on Endocarditis (SEI). BMC Infectious Diseases. 2014;**14**:230

[26] DiNubile MJ, Calderwood SB, Steinhaus DM, Karchmer AW. Cardiacconduction abnormalities complicating native valve active infective endocarditis. The

American Journal of Cardiology. 1986;**58**:1213-1217

[27] Nadji G, Rusinaru D, Remadi JP, Jeu A, Sore lC, Tribouilloy C. Heart failure in left sided native valve infective endocarditis: Characteristics, prognosis, and results of surgical treatment. European Journal of Heart Failure. 2009;**11**:668-675

[28] Hasbun R, Vikram HR, Barakat LA, Buenconsejo J, Quagliarello VJ. Complicated left-sided native valve endocarditis in adults: Risk classification for mortality. JAMA. 2003;**289**:1933-1940

[29] Tornos P, Iung B, Permanyer-Miralda G, Baron G, Delahaye F, GohlkeBarwolf C, et al. Infective endocarditis in Europe: Lessons from the Euro heart survey. Heart. 2005;**91**:571-575

Chapter 6

Aortic Stenosis in Dogs and Cats: Past, Present and Future

Aleksandra Domanjko Petrič, Anja Perovič, Tanja Švara and Peter Dovč

Abstract

Aortic stenosis is one of the three most common congenital heart defects in dogs and less frequent in cats. Most dogs or cats have subvalvular type of stenosis; valvular or supravalvular types are less frequent. Heart failure is seldom a consequence of aortic stenosis; most dogs with heart failure have a concurrent disease. The most common accompanying diagnosis is pulmonic stenosis, especially in the Boxer breed. Screening programs seem to have efficiently lowered the incidence of aortic stenosis in dogs. Genetic evidence for aortic stenosis has been shown in Golden Retriever, Newfoundland and Dogue de Bordeaux; however, the genetic background of aortic stenosis at molecular level remains unclear.

Keywords: aortic stenosis, congenital heart defect, genetics, sudden death, dog, cat

1. Introduction

Aortic stenosis can be defined as a narrowing of the left ventricular outflow tract (LVOT) and/or aorta at the level below the aortic valve, at the aortic valve, or above it. This narrowing produces a blood flow turbulence that is auscultated as a systolic murmur at the heart base, as well as increased blood flow velocity that can be detected and measured by Doppler echocardiography.

Aortic stenosis is mainly considered to be a congenital defect found in many species including humans. In dogs, aortic stenosis has autosomal inheritance; however, the mode of inheritance seems to be more complex in monogenic traits.

Various forms of aortic stenosis as well as its possible genetic background have been recorded in domestic animals since the late 1960s and 1970s [1]. In those times, the final diagnosis was mostly confirmed at necropsy. Currently, diagnosis is based on echocardiographic evaluation of the morphology of the left ventricular outflow tract and aorta and the velocity of blood measured by the continuous wave (CW) Doppler method after a murmur is detected. Prognosis depends on the severity of the stenosis being from no effect on life quality and expectancy in mild forms of the disease to decreased life quality and expectancy in moderate to severe forms due to possible complications. Those include syncopal episodes that can result in sudden death, tiredness on exertion, or in rare cases, congestive heart failure or infective endocarditis [2].

The aim of this chapter is a review of the existing literature and our experience with clinical aspects of AS in dogs and cats. Genetic evidence for aortic stenosis has been shown in Golden Retriever, Newfoundland, and Dogue de Bordeaux; however, the genetic background of aortic stenosis at a molecular level remains unclear.

IntechOpen

2. Forms of aortic stenosis

Subaortic stenosis (SAS) is common congenital cardiac defect in dogs [3, 4] and pigs [5]. In cats, SAS has not been so often described [1, 6–8].

Several classifications are used for aortic stenosis. According to anatomic location, aortic stenosis is classified into valvular (VAS), subvalvular (SAS), or supravalvular (SupAS) [9].

Based on functional characteristics of obstruction, subvalvular cases are further categorized as either fixed (static) or dynamic (labile) [2].

A dynamic form of subaortic stenosis can occur in the following instances: in a hypertrophied left ventricle (LVH) due to protrusion of the ventricular septum into the LVOT, systolic anterior movement of the anterior mitral valve leaflet (SAM) which occurs concurrently or in the absence of LVH, and in cases where aortoseptal angle is smaller than 180° [10].

The subvalvular form—subaortic stenosis (SAS)—has been reported as the most frequently seen (in 95%) and can be presented as a complete or incomplete ring [1, 2, 11–13].

3. Pathologic findings

The gross appearance of the lesions in SAS is variable [4, 14]. Current classification which is used by clinicians is based on anatomical and echocardiographic classification of SAS on the result of postmortem and angiographic studies of Pyle et al. [14, 15]. In a postmortem study performed on Newfoundland puppies, the gross lesions were classified according to severity with grades 1 through 3 [14]. Mild lesions (grade 1) are present as small (1–2 mm), raised white nodules on the endocardium of the ventricular septum below the aortic valve. In some dogs, the nodules are also found on the ventricular surfaces of the aortic valve cusps (**Figure 1**) [14].

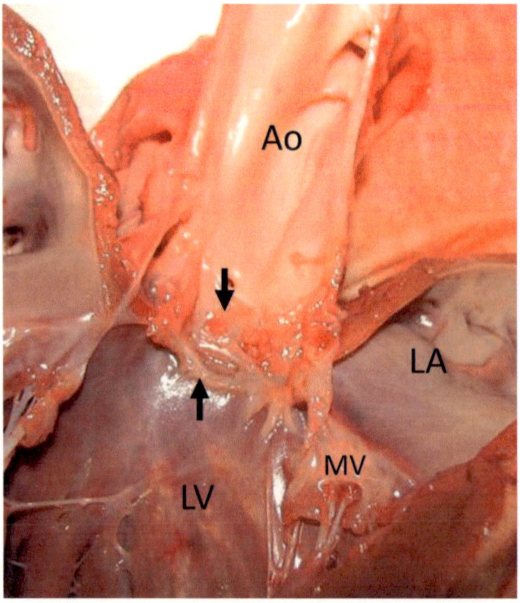

Figure 1.
Gross pathologic specimen from a dog with severe subaortic stenosis. A subvalvular fibrous ring (lower arrow) below the aortic valve and a thickened valve above the fibrous ring of tissue can be seen. Ao—aorta, LV—left ventricle, LA—left atrium, and MV—mitral valve.

Moderate lesions are present as a ridge of endocardial fibrous tissue that in most cases extends from the base of the anterior leaflet of mitral valve across the interventricular septum to beneath the aortic valve (**Figures 2** and **3**) [14]. In severe cases

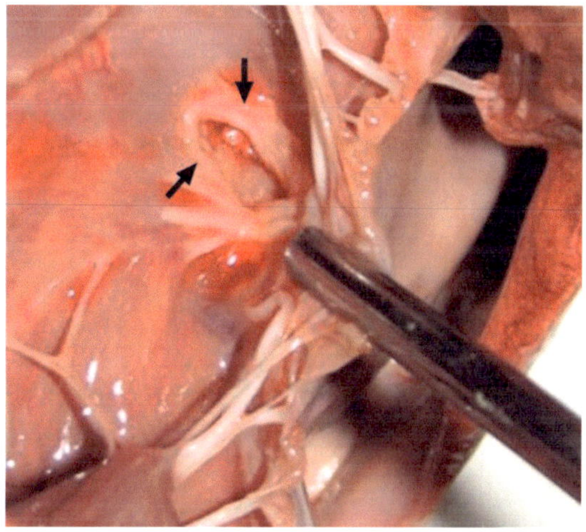

Figure 2.
Gross pathologic specimen from a dog with severe subaortic stenosis. This is a close-up of a closed fibrous subaortic tissue that encircles the left ventricular outflow tract just below the entrance to the aorta.

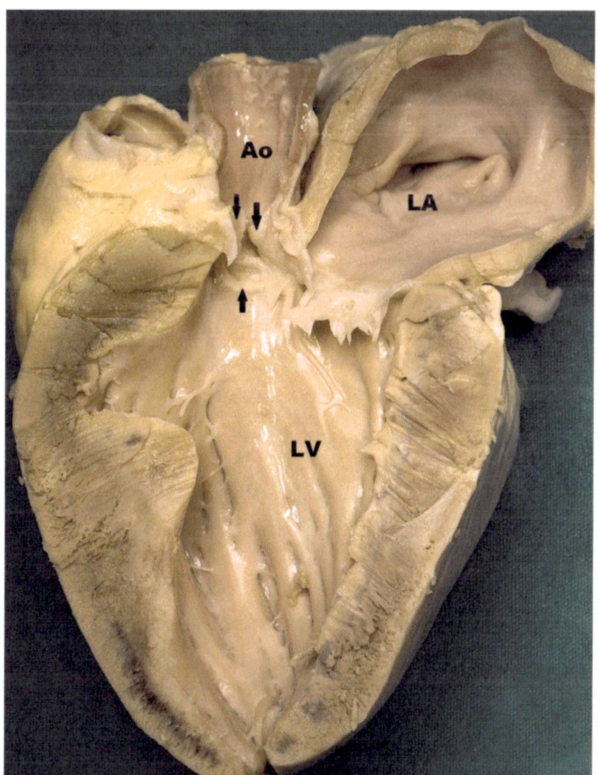

Figure 3.
Gross pathologic specimen from a dog with severe subaortic stenosis. A tunnel-like subaortic stenosis (upper 2 arrows) and a fibrous subaortic ring below the aortic valve is seen (lower arrow). Ao—aorta, LV—left ventricle, and LA—left atrium.

(grade 3), the fibrous band or ridge completely encircles the left ventricular outflow tract below the aortic valve and forms a concentrically narrowing tunnel (**Figure 3**). In most severe cases, anterior leaflet of the mitral valve and ventricular surfaces of the aortic valve are also thickened (**Figure 3**) [14].

Microscopically, the zone of endocardial fibrous tissue below aortic valve contains proliferated mesenchymal cells, mucopolysaccharide ground substance, and foci of metaplastic cartilage [3, 4, 14].

Other cardiac lesions that develop as the consequences of the altered left ventricular outflow include compensatory left ventricular concentric hypertrophy [3] (**Figure 3**) and poststenotic dilatation of the aorta [4].

Microscopic cardiac lesions also include foci of myocardial necrosis, fibrosis in the papillary muscles and subendocardium, thickening of the intramyocardial arteries [3], intimal proliferation of connective tissue, fibrous replacement of smooth muscle in the tunica media [16, 17], and luminal narrowing of intramural coronary arteries [18].

Several cardiac defects have been observed concomitantly with SAS in dogs. These defects include pulmonary artery stenosis (PS), patent ductus arteriosus, mitral valve dysplasia, ventricular septal defect, valvular aortic stenosis, aortic root hypoplasia, persistent left cranial vena cava, bicuspid aorta, quadricuspid aorta, tricuspid dysplasia, double chambered right ventricle, and supravalvular aortic stenosis [19, 20]. Coexistence of aortic stenosis and pulmonary artery stenosis is one of the most common complex cardiac malformations [13, 20].

4. Breed prevalence and natural history

SAS has been ranked the most common congenital heart disease (CHD) in dogs in most European studies accounting for 35% of all CHD. In the United States [12] and in a broad Italian study [20], SAS was on the second place (the most common being PS). However, these results must be taken carefully due to referral population included since a lot of cases were sent for ballooning. Of 4480 dogs included in this study, 976 dogs were diagnosed with congenital heart disease (CHD) of which 21.3% had subaortic stenosis (SAS), while valvular aortic stenosis (AS) was on the fifth place with 5.7% dogs diagnosed. The same study showed many multiple heart defects; the most frequent combination was SAS and PS (26.4%).

We did a study on 9236 dogs, where cardiovascular disease was diagnosed in 6% of dogs, and from those, 12% represented congenital heart diseases of which 45% were aortic stenosis cases [21].

According to many epidemiological studies [20, 22–27], affected breeds are: Boxers, German Shepherd, Newfoundland, Rottweiler, Golden Retriever, Pug, and Bouviers de Flandres. In the Italian study [20] and a Danish study [28], Dogue de Bordeaux was also shown to be significantly affected. German Boxers have proved to be the most sensitive breed in recent years [19, 21, 29–31]. Almost half of all the dogs in the Italian study diagnosed with SAS were Boxers. Boxers are also on top of the list of dogs with pulmonary artery stenosis (PS) and valvular aortic stenosis (AS). In Boxer breed, more male than female dogs are affected with SAS [20, 32]. Studies in cats did not show any breed predilection; aortic stenosis could be of all types described in dogs, with subvalvular stenosis being the most common [6–8, 33]. In our clinic, occasionally a cat with a fixed SAS is detected, usually due to an auscultated murmur. Dynamic left ventricular outflow tract stenosis is much more common in cats due to common occurrence of hypertrophic cardiomyopathy and systolic anterior motion of the mitral valve (personal unpublished data).

Dogs with mild SAS live longer and mostly remain asymptomatic. Prognosis for the untreated condition in this group is good. Dogs with moderate and severe gradients have shorter life expectancy. They have increased risk of infective endocarditis. The majority of dogs with severe gradients (>80 mm Hg) die before 3 years of age. Median survival was 18.9 months [9, 26].

Subaortic stenosis can be a progressive disease that attains its maximal severity within the first 12–15 months [15]. In dogs that already have high aortic velocity, further progression is unlikely; however, dogs with mild stenosis might progress to a moderate stage [34]. Breeding studies also indicate that AS may not be present at birth but develops during the first 4–8 weeks of life, which suggests that AS is not a true congenital trait but develops postnatally [27].

The etiology of SAS is probably multi-factorial [35]. In the literature, there are two hypotheses on how the fibrocartilaginous ring around the LVOT is formed. It could be derived from embryonal endocardial tissue that retains its proliferative capacity and has chondrogenic potential for some time after birth [14]. A more recent hypothesis suggests that certain anatomic characteristics of the LVOT, including an increased mitral-aortic separation, a decreased aortoseptal angle (AoSA), and a small aortic annulus may cause cellular proliferation in the LVOT because of shear stress caused by abnormal flow patterns [35, 36].

Clinical signs such as weakness, syncope, and sudden death are more commonly seen in dogs with severe or moderate AS than in those with mild SAS [2, 9, 11]. Dogs with mild AS rarely show any signs at all [2, 37]. Careful physical examination reveals crescendo-decrescendo systolic murmur from grades 1 to 6. Final diagnosis has to be confirmed by two-dimensional and Doppler echocardiography, by which evaluation of morphologic characteristics, the type of stenosis, and the pressure gradient across the stenosis can be assessed [2, 11, 15].

Cats are more often identified when clinical signs such as heart failure develop [38].

5. Screening schemes

In the early years of the 21th century, cardiac screening programs have been proposed due to high incidence of some congenital heart diseases. Aortic stenosis has been recognized as one of the most common heart defects according to high prevalence in breeds such as Newfoundland dogs, German Boxer, Golden Retrievers, and Rottweiler to name just the ones mostly affected. Therefore, screening programs were introduced to reduce the high prevalence among the breeding dogs. Some breeders became aware that these breeding programs could help to reduce the incidence of affected animals and to breed healthy puppies. In Italy, such a breeding program helped to reduce the high incidence of AS among boxers [32]. In the case of AS, screening involves careful auscultation to detect cardiac murmur, which is a hallmark of AS. In cases where murmurs are found, 2-D and Doppler echocardiography is carried out, where the morphology of the left ventricular outflow tract with the ascending aorta, specific lesions characteristic for AS/SAS, and increased velocity of the aortic flow can be identified [39].

For a screening program to be effective, a good mutual relationship between the veterinarians involved in screening and pertinent kennel clubs need to be established. Kennel club committees responsible for breeding need to suggest to breeders to screen their sires and dams before breeding or define the screening as a condition for breeding into their rulebook.

6. Pathophysiology of aortic stenosis

Stenosis across the left ventricular outflow tract into aorta produces a pressure gradient between the left ventricle and aorta, and the gradient is inversely proportional to the degree of the stenotic orifice. The resistance to flow through the stenosis produces a rise of pressure in the left ventricle through the systole; increased wall stress results in concentric hypertrophy of the ventricle. The flow through the narrow passage is like when we squeeze the hose with water – the velocity (v) of the flow will increase proportionally to the narrowing. The relationship between the pressure and the flow is described by a simplified Bernoulli equation:

Pressure gradient (PG) = $4v^2$.

The velocity of the flow or the pressure gradient is used to assess the severity of the stenosis; higher the velocity or pressure gradient, the more severe is the stenosis. However, interpretation of PG must be careful in sedated and excited animals, where there is a change in the resistance and flow [2].

Additionally, the left ventricular wall diameter and cross-sectional area of the aortic orifice are both proportional to the stenosis and can be used to assess the severity [40]. In the hypertrophied ventricle, diastolic filling can be impaired which can cause mild left atrial enlargement.

Turbulent and high velocity flow through the aortic orifice can damage the cusps, and aortic insufficiency can occur consequently. Damaged cusps can predispose to infective endocarditis, as well.

Animals with aortic stenosis can develop heart failure, although this scenario rarely occurs. Myocardial failure could be the one of the reasons for heart failure to develop; however, other complications such as aortic or mitral insufficiency can lead to this kind of progression.

Dogs or cats with aortic stenosis can die suddenly or experience syncopal episodes. The cause might be the reflex peripheral vasodilation on exertion and bradycardia; on the other hand, sudden hypoxia due to exertion or subendocardial fibrosis can predispose to fatal arrhythmias that can also lead to fatal fibrillation [2].

Arterial pulse in patients with aortic stenosis can be reduced in amplitude and can have a delayed systolic peak [2].

7. Diagnostics

To make a diagnosis of AS, a thorough auscultation of heart sounds and murmurs should be carried out. Auscultation is the basic diagnostic technique to uncover AS and every clinically important AS will produce an audible murmur. It needs to be performed carefully in a quiet environment with a dog standing still to be able to hear low intensity murmurs. Although the murmur grade is found to correlate with the severity of AS, it is important to detect also low-grade murmurs to identify dogs with heart defects [41]. Early diagnosis of murmurs due to congenital heart defects may enable early intervention, which may substantially affect long-term outcomes [42]. Many healthy boxers tend to have a soft systolic low-grade murmur; in a study of 201 healthy Boxers, the prevalence of 1–3 grade murmurs was 56%. Boxers with murmurs had higher ejection velocities than boxers without murmurs [43] and young boxers may more commonly have functional murmurs that can also cause mild increase in ejection velocity due to the physiologic changes.

It has been hypothesized that young animals have a larger stroke volume compared to the size of the great vessels than do older animals. This can result in an increase in flow velocity producing turbulence, either in the aorta or in the pulmonary artery, and a resultant innocent heart murmur. The increase in the velocity and associated turbulence is usually mild, so the heart murmur is soft (i.e., grade 1–3/6). The innocent heart murmur generally disappears before 4 to 6 months of age, when the great vessels enlarge in diameter with growth. A notable exception is the Boxer breed, where a smaller left ventricular outflow tract is associated with systolic murmurs in otherwise normal adults [44].

Aortic or subaortic stenosis produces a typical crescendo-decrescendo mid-systolic to holosystolic murmur heard best over the left heart base or also on the right side of the thorax. Loud murmurs tend to radiate peripherally, some can be heard over the carotid artery or over the head. Severe cases of AS have usually harsh, mixed-frequency murmurs of high grade on the scale from 1 to 6 [41]. Murmur intensity significantly correlates with aortic ejection velocity [13, 41, 45]. Identification of low-intensity murmurs correlates with the level of experience. A stress test increased murmur duration and aortic flow velocity [46]. Assessment of the duration of murmur frequency >200 Hz can be used to distinguish physiologic heart murmurs from murmurs caused by mild AS in Boxers and can be used as a complementary method [47].

8. Electrocardiography

Dogs with mild-to-moderate AS usually produce a normal electrocardiogram on the standard ECG recordings, whereas cases with severe AS may show signs of LV hypertrophy in leads II, III, aVF, V2, and V4. Hypertrophied ventricle can be hypoxic; therefore, depression of the ST segment and T wave changes suggest myocardial ischemia or secondary repolarization changes. We may observe ventricular premature complexes in severe cases as well [45]. In cases where AS is combined with other defects, for example, pulmonic stenosis or tricuspid dysplasia, a right axis deviation might occur, depending on the severity of additional lesions. In our study, in boxers with AS/SAS, arrhythmias were observed in 21% of dogs, such as ventricular premature contractions, left bundle branch block and supraventricular tachycardia, atrial fibrillation, atrial premature contractions, sinus bradycardia, and ventricular preexcitation. Dogs with multiple arrhythmias have ussually also heart failure and/or have concurrent malformations [13]. Holter recordings are recommended in symptomatic dogs for detection of possible arrhythmias or S-T segment changes [2].

9. Echocardiography

Echocardiography is the main noninvasive method for diagnosis of aortic stenosis. Two-dimensional mode is used to detect morphologic abnormalities associated with AS/SAS or supravalvular form. In severe cases, LV concentric hypertrophy, subendocardial hyperechogenicity, representing fibrosis (**Figure 4**), and a small subaortic cross-sectional area (**Figure 5**), is found with 2-D echocardiography. Left ventricular hypertrophy, demonstrated by M-mode, has a positive relationship with disease severity [40]. Subaortic fibrous hyperechogenic tissue protruding into the LVOT is seen in the right parasternal or left parasternal long-axis views (**Figure 6** & https://www.vf.uni-lj.si/izobrazevanje/aortic-stenosis-dogs-and-cats-past-present-and-future). In most cases, some aortic valve thickening can be seen

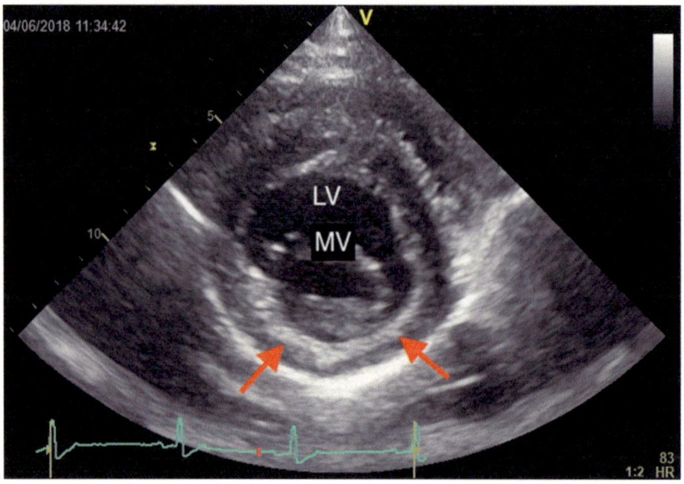

Figure 4.
Two-dimensional echocardiographic image of a short axis of the left ventricle (LV), showing subendocardial fibrosis in the left ventricular free wall. MV—Mitral valve.

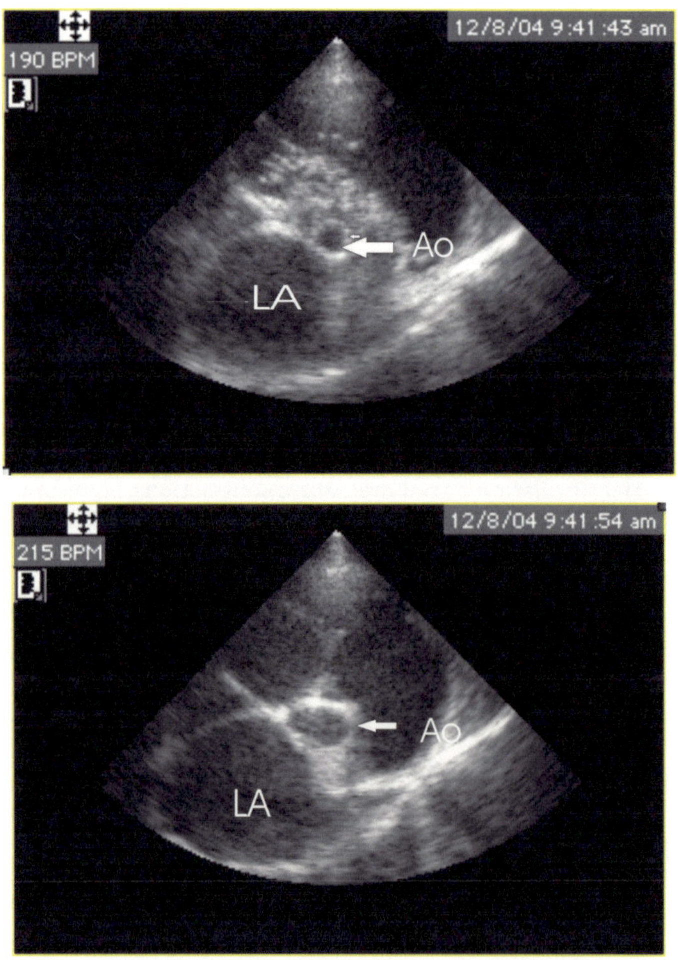

Figure 5.
Two-dimensional echocardiographic image of a short axis at the base of the heart showing subvalvular (upper image) and valvular region (lower image) of the aorta (Ao). One can appreciate the small subvalvular circle compared to the bigger valvular circle. LA—Left atrium.

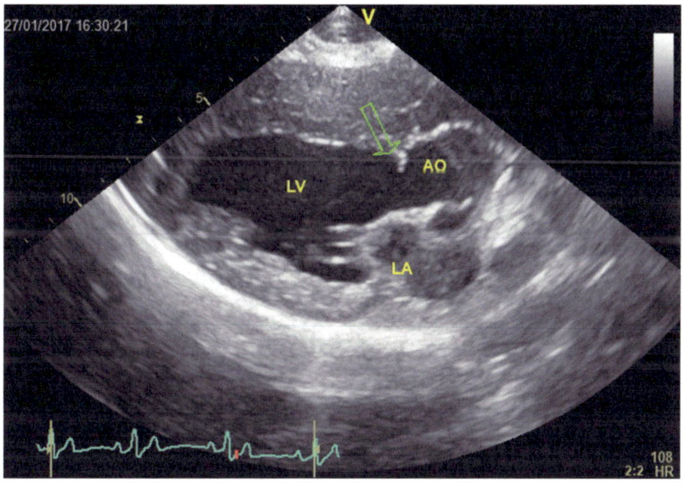

Figure 6.
Subaortic fibrous hyperechogenic tissue protruding into the LVOT is seen in the right parasternal view in a young Newfoundland with severe subaortic stenosis. Ao—aorta, LV—left ventricle, and LA—left atrium.

due to high velocity jets coming to aorta. In cases of true valvular types of stenosis, a poorly moving valve, which does not open completely, can be seen in long-axis (https://www.vf.uni-lj.si/izobrazevanje/aortic-stenosis-dogs-and-cats-past-present-and-future) and cross-sectional views. Color-Doppler mode shows turbulent flow from the obstruction into the aorta (**Figure 7** & https://www.vf.uni-lj.si/izobrazevanje/aortic-stenosis-dogs-and-cats-past-present-and-future). Spectral Doppler modes (continuous Doppler, CW) show high velocity jet, often accompanied with aortic regurgitation (**Figure 8**, https://www.vf.uni-lj.si/izobrazevanje/aortic-stenosis-dogs-and-cats-past-present-and-future). Subcostal transducer placement proved to be superior to the left ventricular apical and the suprasternal view to detect the highest velocity through the aortic orifice [48]. Normal velocities through the aorta differ among breeds and studies; however, the average velocity does not exceed 1.8 m/s from the left apical view or 2 m/s from the subcostal view

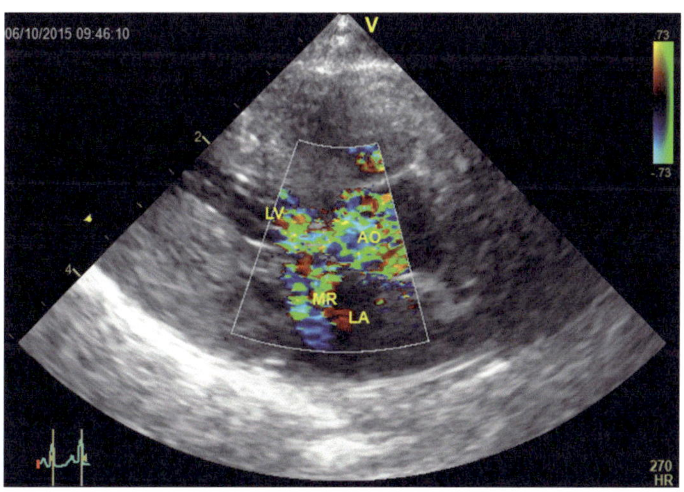

Figure 7.
A color-Doppler flow image of a Sphynx cat with fixed and dynamic subaortic stenosis and concentric hypertrophy of the left ventricle (LV) with concurrent mitral regurgitation (MR).

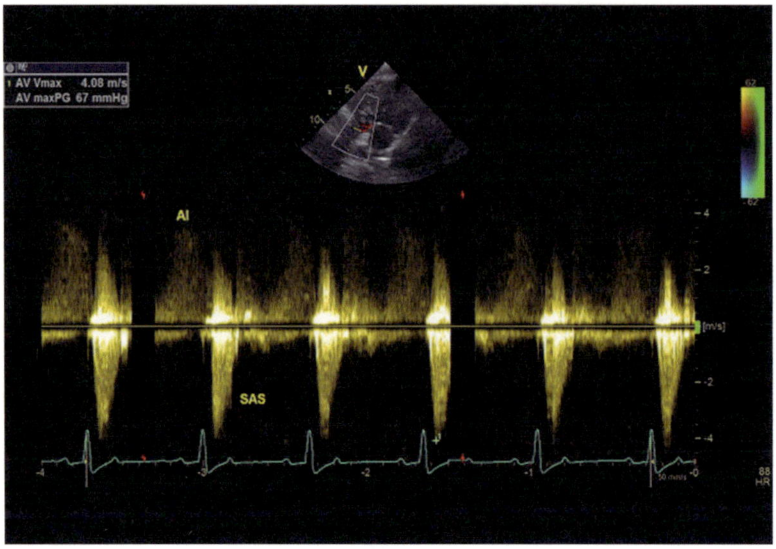

Figure 8.
Continuous wave Doppler across the aortic orifice showing a high velocity jet (AS) of 4 m/s below the baseline, which gives a pressure gradient of 67 mmHg and an aortic insufficiency jet in diastole above the baseline(AI).

[49]. In Boxers without murmurs, higher normal velocities are reported, that is, 2.38 m/s due to smaller LVOT [43, 50].

It is important to use low-frequency transducer for Doppler studies to ensure good penetration of tissues and adequate signal strength to obtain good flow recordings of maximal velocities. Diagnostic problem represents dogs with low intensity murmurs and subtle echocardiographic changes. No association was found between heart rate and aortic velocity [41].

Aortic stenosis has been graded as "mild," with pressure gradients (PG) either from 16 to 40 mmHg (corresponding to aortic velocities, (v), of 2.0–3.16 m/sec) or from 20 to 49 mmHg (corresponding to velocities of 2.25–3.5 m/sec, "moderate," with PG either from 40 to 80 mmHg (v = 3.1.6–4.5 m/sec) or 50 to 80 mmHg (v = 3.5–4.5 m/sec), and "severe" with PG above 80 mmHg, corresponding to velocities over 4.5 m/sec [2, 15]. Pressure gradients derived by Doppler echocardiography showed good agreement with direct pressure measurements, especially for mean gradients [51].

10. Radiography and computed tomography

Thoracic radiographs may appear normal in dogs with AS/SAS; however, in severe cases, LV enlargement may be visible due to LVH and/or post-stenotic dilation of the aortic arch (**Figures 9** and **10**).

In cases where AS is combined with other defects, pertinent radiographic changes may be apparent. Congestive heart failure is rare in SAS, it might be observed in severe cases or with concurrent mitral regurgitation, aortic or mitral endocarditis [2].

Angiographic methods for further evaluation of aortic stenosis morphology are nowadays replaced with contrast computed tomography (CT) scans where needed in terms of interventional or surgical treatment plans. Cardiac CT angiography allows visualization of cardiac chambers and great vessels as well as coronary vessels through cardiac cycles retrospectively. Evaluation of the coronary arteries in the patient is commonly focused on determining if an aberrant vessel is present, which may relate to a pulmonic stenosis, which can be present concurrently with AS/SAS.

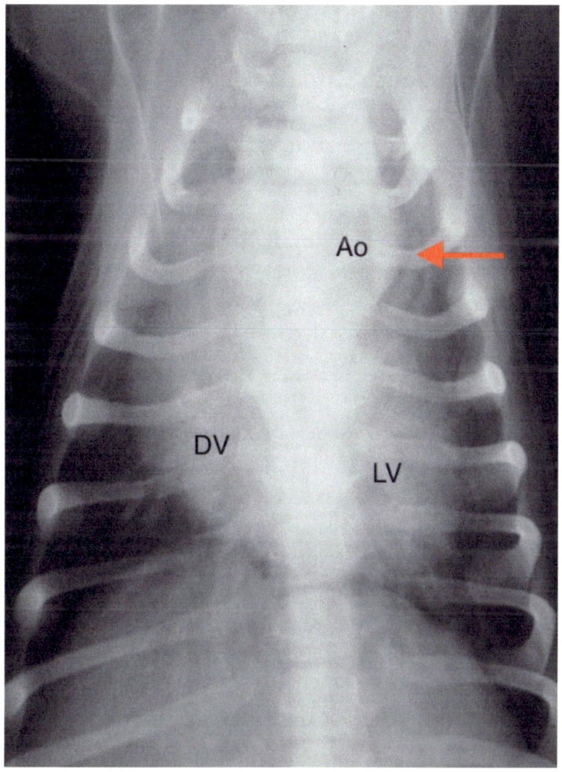

Figure 9.
A dorsoventral thoracic radiograph of a 4-month-old Irish setter with severe aortic stenosis. A post-stenotic dilation of aortic arch is seen (arrow). Ao—aorta, RV—right ventricle, and LV—left ventricle.

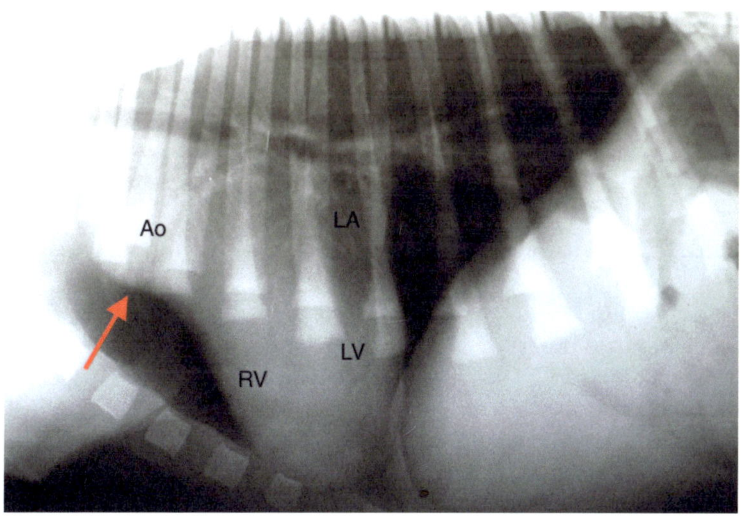

Figure 10.
*A right lateral thoracic radiograph of the same dog as in **Figure 9**, showing a post-stenotic dilation of aortic arch (arrow). DV—right ventricle and LA—left atrium.*

11. Therapeutic possibilities

Prognosis of animals with aortic stenosis depends on the severity of the disease. Mild stenosis usually does not affect longevity; however, the possibility of aortic endocarditis exists, and antibiotic prophylaxis is recommended for dogs and cats with aortic stenosis [52].

Balloon valvuloplasty, although with an average 50% reduction in PG after ballooning, has not proved to be a long-term solution, because in most dogs restenosis occured [53]; however, in some cases, it may reduce clinical signs [54].

No clear benefit in survival times was seen for dogs that underwent balloon valvuloplasty versus dogs that were treated with atenolol [55].

A new technique with a high-pressure ballooning or a cutting balloon might represent an opportunity for better outcome for dogs with AS/SAS, but to date we have no long-term results [56]. Moreover, aortoseptal angle >160° was associated with better long-term outcomes of treated dogs with cutting and high-pressure balloon [57, 58]. Authors and also others recommend saving patients with moderate and severe AS/SAS against strenuous exercise. Administration of beta-blockers can decrease heart rate, prolong diastole and coronary filling, thereby reducing myocardial hypoxia and protect against arrhythmia. Dogs do clinically well on beta-blockers; however, a study proved no benefit in terms of survival versus untreated dogs with severe SAS [59]. There is no literature on evaluation of other medical treatment.

Surgical options such as closed transventricular valvotomy or open-heart surgery can present an option for dogs with symptomatic or severe AS/SAS; however, also these techniques did not provide long-term benefits or prevent sudden death. Additionally, they are not widely available, and they are risky and costly [60–63]. Hopefully, this might change in the future with the development of minimally invasive techniques and their availability in veterinary medicine.

12. Genetic aspects of aortic stenosis

Comparison of mixed and pure-breed dog populations showed a tendency toward higher incidence of AS in pure-breed dog populations [64]. Among pure-breed dogs, the incidence of AS is increased in herding, working, sporting, mastiff-like, and retriever breeds. The fact that the higher incidence of AS is associated with the increase of inbreeding coefficient in the population supports the suggestion that AS has a genetic component. Online Mendelian Inheritance in Animals (OMIA) database also reports AS in dog as heritable disorder with unclear mode of inheritance [65].

12.1 Evidence for genetic background

Genetic background of AS has been studied in several dog breeds with the aim to decipher its mode of inheritance and causal mutation for it. In the Dogue de Bordeaux, association of AS with several physiological parameters as left-basilar ejection murmur, increased aortic ejection velocity, smaller aortic annulus and decreased aortoseptal angle was discovered and genetic predisposition for AS in Dogue de Bordeaux has been proposed [28]. Familial nature of subvalvular aortic stenosis (SAS) was discovered in Golden retrievers [66] based on pedigree data, where SAS has been observed in several subsequent generations. Although a bit controversial, the most complete data about the genetic base of AS are available for Newfoundland dogs. In the study performed by Reist-Marti [67], an extensive pedigree data set comprising more than 230,000 Newfoundland dogs from European and North American population reaching back to the 19th century has been investigated. Similar to the situation in Golden retrievers, the autosomal inheritance was proposed. In addition, statistically significant association between the inbreeding level and incidence of SAS was also found. However, the most precise information about the putative molecular background of AS in Newfoundland dogs was discovered by Stern et al. [68]. The authors propose that a three-nucleotide insertion in the genomic region, coding for phosphatidylinositol-binding clathrin assembly protein (PICalM) is associated with the appearance of AS. The pedigree evaluation, similarly as in Newfoundland dogs, supported an autosomal dominant mode of inheritance. The authors demonstrated the presence of PICalM in the canine myo cardium and in the area of the subvalvular ridge immunohistochemically, which is supporting the assumption that PICalM has a role in development of AS.

In Boxers, AS seems to have a genetic background too; however, the causal locus (loci) has not been identified yet. The higher risk for AS in Boxers might be associated with some breed-specific conformational traits, like small aortic annulus and steep aortoseptal angle [69]. The incomplete penetrance of modifier genes together with autosomal dominant mode of inheritance may be the expected genetic base for AS in Boxers [32].

12.2 Genetic diagnostics

Due to the rapid development of genome analysis in all species, several novel approaches are available also in dog genetics. From the genetic point of view, dog breeds represent a very special taxonomic group, characterized by extremely long regions of linkage disequilibrium (LD) compared to other species. This enables a very effective identification of causal genomic regions associated with monogenic genetic disorders using relatively small groups of animals in case versus control format of studies. The most frequently used strategy in this context is genome-wide association studies (GWAS), which can precisely map location of candidate genes in the genome. The candidate gene regions are then further screened for polymorphic sites using the targeted sequencing strategy in order to find causal mutation for genetic disorder (**Figure 11**). However, complex traits, where a larger number of loci are involved in phenotype shaping, represent a much more difficult task and normally require a larger number of individuals for genetic studies.

12.3 Advices for breeding in the future

The number of registered inherited disorders in dogs is permanently growing (over 400 disorders), and in many dog breeds, the point is reached where for the

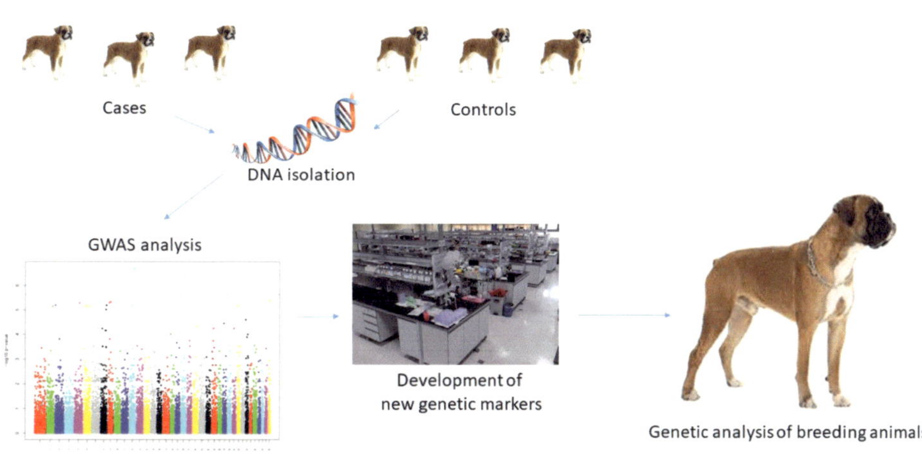

Figure 11.
Summary of development and application of genetic markers for diagnosis of hereditary diseases.

successful breeding against spreading genetic disorders within the breed requires new strategies in combination with currently available breeding schemes. The widespread use of a popular sire caused the overrepresentation of genomes of a low number of sires in many breeds. As a consequence, the effective population size reduced drastically and the risk for rapid dissemination of monogenic disorders within the population increased significantly. The accessibility of reliable genetic tests for detection of carriers of recessive disease-associated alleles represents an important tool for reduction or even elimination of genetic disorders from pure-breed populations. Increasing the number of breeding animals (especially males), controlled introgression of genetic material into closed pure-breed populations, and application of advanced breeding strategies are measures, which will help the breeders to keep genetic pools of different dog breeds healthy.

13. Future perspectives and conclusions

Aortic/subaortic stenosis has a guarded prognosis if moderate to severe; however, efforts have been made in several aspects to fight the disease. First, screening programs have lowered the incidence of the disease (Bussadori 2006, personal unpublished data), and secondly, interventional methods have advanced and might give better prognosis for severely affected dogs; on the other hand, there is still room for surgical methods to take place in veterinary medicine and be more readily available. The genetic background for aortic stenosis is not completely known; however, several mutations, associated with the disease in different breeds, allow development of strategies for genetic screening which would reduce the risk for the disease in pure-breed dogs.

Acknowledgements

The authors acknowledge the financial support of the Slovenian Research Agency (research programs P4-0053 and P4-0092).

Conflict of interest

The authors have no conflicts of interest to disclose.

Author details

Aleksandra Domanjko Petrič[1]*, Anja Perovič[2], Tanja Švara[3] and Peter Dovč[4]

1 Small Animal Clinic, Veterinary Faculty, University of Ljubljana, Ljubljana, Slovenia

2 Sonar d.o.o., Ljubljana, Slovenia

3 Institute of Pathology, Wild Animals, Fish and Bees, Veterinary Faculty University of Ljubljana, Ljubljana, Slovenia

4 Biotechnical Faculty, Department of Animal Science, University of Ljubljana, Domžale, Slovenia

*Address all correspondence to: aleksandra.domanjko@vf.uni-lj.si

References

[1] King JM, Flint TJ, Anderson WI. Incomplete subaortic stenotic rings in domestic animals—A newly described congenital anomaly. The Cornell Veterinarian. 1988;**78**:263-271

[2] Kienle RK. Aortic stenosis. In: Kittleson MD, Kienle RD. Small Animal Cardiovascular Medicine. 1st ed. Maryland Heights, Missouri: Mosby; 1998: 260-272

[3] Miller LM, Van Vleet JF, Cardiovascular System GA, Vessels L. In: Zachary JF, McGavin MD, editors. Pathologic Basis of Veterinary Disease. 5th ed. St. Louis, Missouri: Elsevier Mosby; 2012. pp. 539-589

[4] Robinson WF, Robinson NA. Cardiovascular system. In: Grant Maxie M, editor. Jubb, Kennedy, and Palmer's Pathology of Domestic Animals. 6th ed. Philadelphia, PA: Elsevier Saunders; 2016. pp. 2-22. DOI: 10.1016/C2012-0-00823-X

[5] Hsu FS, Du SJ. Congenital heart diseases in swine. Veterinary Pathology. 1982;**19**:676-686. DOI: 10.1177/030098588201900613

[6] Margiocco ML, Zini E. Fixed subaortic stenosis in a cat. The Veterinary Record. 2005;**156**:712-714

[7] Sousa MG, Pascon JP, de Brum AM, Santos PAC, Camacho AA. Severe aortic stenosis in a Persian kitten. RPCV. 2008;**103**:229-232

[8] Ferreira AM, Stedile STO, Silva VBC, Souza MG. Arterial thromboembolism secondary to subaortic stenosis in a Persian kitten. Acta Scientiae Veterinariae. 2018;**46**(Suppl 1):292

[9] Kienle RD, Thomas WP, Pion PD. The natural clinical history of canine congenital subaortic stenosis. Journal of Veterinary Internal Medicine/American College of Veterinary Internal Medicine. 1994;**8**:423-431

[10] Zuluaga Santamaría A, Aldana SN, Gutiérrez MC, Bustamante ZS, Muñoz C, GP ZMN. Left ventricular outflow tract obstruction. The Revista Colombiana de Entomología. 2017;**28**(1):4609-4615

[11] O'Grady MR, Holmberg DL, Miller CW, et al. Canine congenital aortic stenosis: A review of the literature and commentary. The Canadian Veterinary Journal/La Revue Vétérinaire Canadienne. 1989;**30**:811

[12] Buchanan JW. Prevalence of cardiovascular disorders. In: Fox PR, Sisson DD, Moise NS, editors. Textbook of Canine and Feline Cardiology. 2nd ed. Philadelphia, PA: WB Saunders Company; 1999. pp. 458-463

[13] Domanjko-Petrič A, Cvetko S. Aortic stenosis in dogs: Clinical characteristics and survival in 80 cases. Slovenian Veterinary Research. 2009;**46**:125-131

[14] Pyle RL, Patterson DF, Chacko S. The genetics and pathology of discrete subaortic stenosis in the Newfoundland dog. American Heart Journal. 1976;**92**:324-334

[15] Bussadori C, Amberger C, Le Bobinnec G, et al. Guidelines for the echocardiographic studies of suspected subaortic stenosis. Journal of Veterinary Cardiology: The official journal of the European Society of Veterinary Cardiology. 2000;**2**:15-22. DOI: 10.1016/S1760-2734(06)70007-8

[16] Flickinger GL, Patterson DF. Coronary lesions associated with congenital subaortic stenosis in the dog. The Journal of Pathology and Bacteriology. 1967;**93**:133-140. DOI: 10.1002/path.1700930113

[17] Freedom RM, Yoo SJ, Russell J, Perrin D, Williams WG. Thoughts about

fixed subaortic stenosis in man and dog. Cardiology in the Young. 2005;**15**:186-205. DOI: 10.1017/S1047951105000399

[18] Falk T, Jönsson L, Pedersen HD. Intramyocardial arteries narrowing in dogs with subaortic stenosis. The Journal of Small Animal Practice. 2004;**45**:448-453

[19] Tidholm A. Retrospective study of congenital heart defects in 151 dogs. The Journal of Small Animal Practice. 1997;**38**:94-98

[20] Oliveira P, Domenech O, Silva J, Vannini S, Bussadori R, Bussadori C. Retrospective review of congenital heart disease in 976 dogs. Journal of Veterinary Internal Medicine/ American College of Veterinary Internal Medicine. 2011;**25**:477-483. DOI: 10.1111/j.1939-1676.2011.0711.x

[21] Domanjko Petric A, Hozjan E. Epidemiological study of cardiovascular diseases in Slovenia. In: Proceedings of ECVIM Barcelona. 2004. p. 212

[22] Detweiler DK, Patterson DF. The prevalence and types of cardiovascular disease in dogs. Annals of the New York Academy of Sciences. 1965;**127**:481-516

[23] Detweiler DK, Hubben K, Patterson DF. Survey of cardiovascular disease in dogs: Preliminary report on the first 1000 dogs screened. American Journal of Veterinary Research. 1960;**21**:329-359

[24] Fernandez del Palacio MJ, Bayon A, Bernal LJ, Ceron JJ, Navarro JA. Clinical and pathological findings of severe subvalvular aortic stenosis and mitral dysplasia in a rottweiler puppy. The Journal of Small Animal Practice. 1998;**39**:481-485

[25] Patterson DF. Congenital defects of the cardiovascular system of dogs: Studies in comparative cardiology. Advances in Veterinary Science and Comparative Medicine. 1976;**20**:1-37

[26] Patterson DF. Epidemiologic and genetic studies of congenital heart disease in the dog. Circulation Research. 1968;**23**:171-202

[27] Patterson DF. Canine congenital heart disease: Epidemiology and etiological hypotheses. The Journal of Small Animal Practice. 1971;**12**:263-287

[28] Hollmer M. Aortic stenosis in the Dogue de Bordeaux. Journal of Small Animal Practice. 2008;**49**:432-437

[29] Bussadori C, Domenech O, Pradelli D. Canine subaortic stenosis-pathoanatomical observations in Italian boxers. In: Proceedings FECAVA Congres Berlin. 2001. pp. 16-18

[30] Baumgartner C, Glaus TM. Congenital cardiac diseases in dogs: A retrospective analysis. Schweizer Archiv für Tierheilkunde. 2003;**145**:527-536. DOI: 10.1024/0036-7281.145.11.527

[31] Le Bobinnec G. Canine subaortic stenosis: Epidemiology in France, ECG changes, antiarhytmic drug therapy. In: Proceedings FECAVA Congress Berlin. 2001. pp. 12-15

[32] Bussadori C. Congenital heart disease in boxer dogs: Results of 6 years of breed screening. The Veterinary Journal. 2009;**181**:187-192

[33] Zook BC. Some spontaneous Cardiovascular lesions in dogs and cats. In: Comparative pathology of the heart. Symposium, Boston, mass, September 1973. Advances in Cardiology, Basel, Karger. 1974;**13**:148-168. DOI: 10.1159/000395535

[34] French A, Luis Fuentes V, Dukes-McEwan J, Darke PG, Martin M, Corcoran B. Progression of aortic stenosis in the boxer. The Journal of Small Animal Practice. 2000;**41**(10):451-456

[35] Cilliers AM, Gewillig M. Rheology of discrete subaortic stenosis. Heart (British Cardiac Society). 2002;**88**:335-336

[36] Cape EG, Vanauker MD, SigfússonG TTA, Del Nido PJ. Potential role of mechanical stress in the etiology of pediatric heart disease: Septal shear stress in subaortic stenosis. Journal of the American College of Cardiology. 1997;**30**:247-254

[37] Pasławska U, Cepiel A, Noszczyk-Nowak A, Staszczyk M, Janiszewski A. Epidemiological prevalence of aortic stenosis in dogs in Poland. Medycyna Weterynaryjna. 2014;**70**:550-552

[38] Stepien RL, Bonagura JD. Aortic stenosis: Clinical findings in six cats. The Journal of Small Animal Practice. 1991. DOI: 10.1111/j.1748-5827.1991.tb00945.x

[39] Fuentes VL. Methods of screening for subaortic stenosis. In: Proceedings 14th ECVIM Annual Congress, 9-11 September 2004; Barcelona ECVIM-CA. 2004

[40] Oyama MA, Thomas WP. Two-dimensional and M-mode echocardiographic predictors of disease severity in dogs with congenital subaortic stenosis. Journal of the American Animal Hospital Association. 2002;**38**(3):209-215. DOI: 10.5326/0380209

[41] Kvart C, French AT, Fuentes VL, Häggström J, McEwan JD, Schober KE. Analysis of murmur intensity, duration and frequency components in dogs with aortic stenosis. The Journal of Small Animal Practice. 1998;**39**(7):318-324

[42] Bélanger M-C, Côté E. In: Ettinger SJ, Feldman EC, editors. Innocent Heart Murmurs. 7th ed. Philadelphia: Saunders; 2010. pp. 256-259

[43] Koplitz SL, Meurs KM, Spier AW, Bonagura JD, Fuentes VL, Wright NA. Aortic ejection velocity in healthy boxers with soft cardiac murmurs and boxers without cardiac murmurs: 201 cases (1997-2001). Journal of the American Veterinary Medical Association. 2003;**222**(6):770-774

[44] Koplitz SL, Meurs KM, Bonagura JD. Echocardiographic assessment of the left ventricular outflow tract in the boxer. Journal of Veterinary Internal Medicine/American College of Veterinary Internal Medicine. 2006;**20**(4):904-911

[45] Linde A, Koch J. Screening for aortic stenosis in the boxer: Auscultatory, ECG, blood pressure and Doppler echocardiographic findings. Journal of Veterinary Cardiology. 2006;**8**:79-86. DOI: 10.1016/j.jvc.2006.02.002

[46] Höglund K, French A, Dukes-McEwan J, Häggström J, Smith P, Corcoran B, et al. Low intensity heart murmurs in boxer dogs: Inter-observer variation and effects of stress testing. The Journal of Small Animal Practice. 2004;**45**(4):178-185

[47] Höglund K, Ahlstrom CH, Häggström J, Ask PN, Hult PH, Kvart C. Time-frequency and complexity analyses for differentiation of physiologic murmurs from heart murmurs caused by aortic stenosis in boxers. American Journal of Veterinary Research. 2007;**68**(9):962-969

[48] Lehmkuhl LB, Bonagura JD. Comparison of transducer placement sites for Doppler echocardiography in dogs with subaortic stenosis. American Journal of Veterinary Research. 1994;**55**(2):192-198

[49] Beijerink NJ, Oyama AM, Bonagura JD. Congenital Heart Disease. In: Ettinger SJ, Feldman, EC, Cote, E. eds. 8th ed. Philadelphia: Saunders; 2017. p 1235-1240

[50] Schober KE, Fuentes VL. Doppler echocardiographic assessment of

left ventricular diastolic function in 74 boxer dogs with aortic stenosis. Journal of Veterinary Cardiology. 2002;**4**(1):7-16. DOI: 10.1016/S1760-2734(06)70018-2

[51] Lehmkuhl LB, Bonagura JD, Jones DE, Stepien RL. Comparison of catheterization and Doppler-derived pressure gradients in a canine model of subaortic stenosis. Journal of the American Society of Echocardiography: Official Publication of the American Society of Echocardiography. 1995;**8** (5 Pt 1):611-620

[52] Roth L. Bacterial aortic valvular endocarditis associated with subvalvular aortic stenosis. The Journal of Small Animal Practice. 1994;**35**:169-172. DOI: https://doi.org/10.1111/j.1748-5827.1994.tb03924

[53] DeLellis LA, Thomas WP, Pion PD. Balloon dilation of congenital subaortic stenosis in the dog. Journal of Veterinary Internal Medicine/American College of Veterinary Internal Medicine. 1993;7(3):153-162

[54] Han SW, Lee CM, Park HM. Balloon valvuloplasty for severe subaortic stenosis in a Pomeranian dog. Korean Journal of Veterinary Research. 2016;**56**(4):261-264. DOI: 10.14405/kjvr.2016.56.4.261

[55] Meurs KM, Lehmkuhl LB, Bonagura JD. Survival times in dogs with severe subvalvular aortic stenosis treated with balloon valvuloplasty or atenolol. Journal of the American Veterinary Medical Association. 2005;**227**(3):420-424

[56] Kleman ME, Estrada AH, Maisenbacher HW 3rd, Prošek R, Pogue B, Shih A, et al. How to perform combined cutting balloon and high pressure balloon valvuloplasty for dogs with subaortic stenosis. Journal of veterinary Cardiology: The Official Journal of the European Society of Veterinary Cardiology. 2012;**14**(2):351-361. DOI: 10.1016/j.jvc.2011.11.008

[57] Shen L, Estrada AH, Côté E, Powell MA, Winter B, Lamb K. Aortoseptal angle and pressure gradient reduction following balloon valvuloplasty in dogs with severe subaortic stenosis. Journal of Veterinary Cardiology. 2017 Apr;**19**(2):144-152. DOI: 10.1016/j.jvc.2016.10.005

[58] Scansen BA. Cardiac interventions in small animals: Areas of uncertainty. Veterinary Clinics of North America Small Animal Practice. Sep 2018;**48**(5):797-817. DOI: 10.1016/j.cvsm.2018.05.003. Epub 2018 Jun 18

[59] Eason BD, Fine DM, Leeder D, Stauthammer C, Lamb K, Tobias AH. Influence of beta blockers on survival in dogs with severe subaortic stenosis. Journal of Veterinary Internal Medicine/American College of Veterinary Internal Medicine. 2014;**28**(3):857-862. DOI: 10.1111/jvim.12339

[60] Komtebedde J, Ilkiw JE, Follette DM, Breznock EM, Tobias AH. Resection of subvalvular aortic stenosis. Surgical and perioperative management in seven dogs. Veterinary Surgery: VS. 1993;**22**(6):419-430

[61] Monnet E, Orton EC, Gaynor JS, Boon J, Wagner A, Linn K, et al. Open resection for subvalvular aortic stenosis in dogs. Journal of the American Veterinary Medical Association. 1996;**209**(7):1255-1261

[62] Linn K, Orton EC. Closed transventricular dilation of discrete subvalvular aortic stenosis in dogs. Veterinary Surgery: VS. 1992;**21**(6):441-445

[63] Dhokarikar P, Caywood DD, Ogburn PN, Stobie D, Burtnick NL. Closed aortic valvotomy: A retrospective study in 15 dogs. Journal of the American Animal Hospital

Association. 1995;**31**(5):402-410. DOI: 10.5326/15473317-31-5-402

[64] Oberbauer AM, Belanger JM, Bellumori T, Bannasch DL, Famula TR. Ten inherited disorders in pure-breed dogs by functional breed groupings. Canine Genetics and Epidemiology. 2015;**2**:9. DOI: 10.1186/s40575-015-0021-x

[65] OMIA 000052-9615: Aortic stenosis, subvalvular in *Canis lupus familiaris* [Internet]. Available from: https://omia.org/OMIA000052/9615/ [Accessed: 15-01-2019]

[66] Stern JA, Meurs KM, Nelson OL, Lahmers SM, Lehmkuhl LB. Familial subvalvular aortic stenosis in golden retrievers: Inheritance and echocardiographic findings. Journal of Small Animal Practice. 2012;**53**:213-216

[67] Reist-Marti SB, Dolf G, Leeb T, Kottmann S, Kietzmann S, Butenhoff K, et al. Genetic evidence of subaortic stenosis in the Newfoundland dog. The Veterinary Record. 2012;**170**(23):597. DOI: 10.1136/vr.100019

[68] JA1 S, White SN, Lehmkuhl LB, Reina-Doreste Y, Ferguson JL, Nascone-Yoder NM, et al. A single codon insertion in PICALM is associated with development of familial subvalvular aortic stenosis in Newfoundland dogs. Human Genetics. 2014;**133**(9):1139-1148. DOI: 10.1007/s00439-014-1454-0

[69] Quintavalla C, Guazzetti S, Mavropoulou A, Bussadori C. Aorto-septal angle in Boxer dogs with subaortic stenosis: An echocardiographic study. Journal of Veterinary Science. Sep 2010;**185**(3):332-337. DOI: 10.1016/j.tvjl.2009.06.027. Epub 2009 Aug 7

Chapter 7

Hemodynamic Classifications of Aortic Stenosis and Relevance to Prognosis

Susan Kwon and Aasha Gopal

Abstract

Hemodynamic classifications of aortic valve stenosis (AS) have important prognostic implications. In normal flow state, severe AS is defined as peak aortic velocity ≥ 4.0 m/s, mean transaortic gradient (MG) ≥ 40 mmHg, and aortic valve area (AVA) < 1.0 cm^2. However, numerous studies have shown that severe AS (based on AVA < 1.0 cm^2) with low gradient (MG < 40 mmHg) is prevalent due to low flow state, in the setting of reduced and preserved left ventricular ejection fraction (LVEF). Thus, the hemodynamic classifications of AS with AVA < 1.0 cm^2 were expanded to include the transvalvular flow state and pressure gradients. These flow-gradient patterns include normal flow/very high gradient, normal flow/high gradient, low flow/high gradient, low flow/low gradient with reduced LVEF, low flow/low gradient with preserved LVEF, and normal flow/low gradient. Among these, the low-gradient AS subgroups are challenging, particularly to differentiate true-severe AS (where aortic valve replacement is necessary) and pseudo-severe AS (where conservative management is recommended). Additional diagnostic studies such as dobutamine stress echocardiography and/or cardiac computed tomography, as well as other parameters such as projected AVA and/or valvuloarterial impedance may be helpful. This chapter will review diagnostic approaches and prognostic implications of different AS subtypes.

Keywords: aortic stenosis, classification, echocardiography, hemodynamics, low flow, prognosis

1. Introduction

Aortic valve stenosis (AS) is the most common valvular heart disease in developed countries. When symptomatic, AS is known to have significant morbidity and mortality. While the prevalence of AS is expected to rise with the aging population, there is no pharmacological treatment option to prevent its progression at this time [1, 2]. Aortic valve replacement (AVR) is the only treatment demonstrated to improve survival and symptoms [3, 4]. Therefore, in the management of patients with AS, it is essential to accurately diagnose the disease severity and determine the proper timing of surgical referral. According to the ACC/AHA guidelines, AVR is class I indication for patients with symptomatic severe AS with high transaortic mean gradient (MG) ≥ 40 mmHg and left ventricular (LV) ejection fraction (LVEF) < 50% and/or who are undergoing another surgery [5]. Over the past decade, challenges due to discrepancies with grading

High Gradient (HG) (MG ≥ 40 mmHg)	Low Gradient (LG) (MG < 40 mmHg)
NF/Very HG Normal Flow (SVI ≥ 35 ml/m^2), (MG > 60 mmHg)	**LF/LG with reduced LVEF** Low Flow (SVI < 35 ml/m2), LVEF < 50%
NF/HG Normal Flow (SVI ≥ 35 ml/m^2)	**LF/LG with preserved LVEF** Low Flow (SVI < 35 ml/m^2), LVEF ≥ 50%
LF/HG Low Flow (SVI < 35 ml/m^2)	**NF/LG** Normal Flow (SVI ≥ 35 ml/m^2)
AVA, aortic valve area; MG, mean transaortic gradient; HG, high gradient; LG, low gradient; NF, normal flow; LF, low flow; SVI, stroke volume index; LVEF, left ventricular ejection fraction.	

Table 1.
Hemodynamic classification of severe aortic stenosis (AVA < 1.0 cm^2).

AS severity and the necessity of integrating the valve gradient with flow patterns were recognized when a significant subset of patients were found to have small AVAs suggestive of severe AS with lower gradients despite preserved LVEF [6]. As a result, under the umbrella of severe AS (based on AVA < 1.0 cm^2), a new hemodynamic classification of AS was proposed which can be categorized into six subgroups based on LV flow state [normal flow (NF) vs. low flow (LF)] and pressure gradient [very high gradient (VHG) vs. high gradient (HG) vs. low gradient (LG)]. These six flow-gradient patterns (NF/VHG, NF/HG, LF/HG, LF/LG with reduced LVEF, LF/LG with preserved LVEF, and normal NF/LG) have shown to represent distinct pathophysiologic types of severe AS with different clinical outcomes (see **Table 1**).

2. Natural history of AS

AS is a progressive valvular heart disease with gradual valvular narrowing resulting in LV outflow tract (LVOT) obstruction over time. Degenerative calcific AS is the most common type of this disease process and predominantly affects the elderly. With this condition, there is a long latent period during which the patient is asymptomatic although there is progression of obstructive physiology at the aortic valve and LV pressure overload. Survival in asymptomatic patients undergoing conservative management with watchful waiting is not statistically different from age- and gender-matched controls [7]. However, once symptoms of angina, syncope, or heart failure develop, there is a very rapid decline. Patients with AS who develop angina have a 5-year survival, syncope 3-year survival, and heart failure, the most ominous of all, 2-year survival (see **Figure 1**) [8, 9]. Thus, when symptoms are corroborated by established echocardiographic criteria for severe AS, some form of intervention is required because these individuals only have a 3-year survival of about 25%. In severe asymptomatic AS, the rate of symptom onset is higher when significant calcification of the aortic valve is present and in older patients [7]. Other factors demonstrated to predict symptom onset and surgical outcome include brain natriuretic peptide (BNP) [10]. While the risk of sudden death is a major concern in patients with asymptomatic AS undergoing conservative management, numerous studies have shown that the risk is very low, <1% per year [7, 11, 12].

Over the years, there has been marked decrease in the operative risk of AS. Furthermore, while prior studies have shown rather benign prognosis of asymptomatic severe AS patients, suggesting that delay in surgery can be safe until the development of symptoms, there is controversy as to the optimal timing of AVR

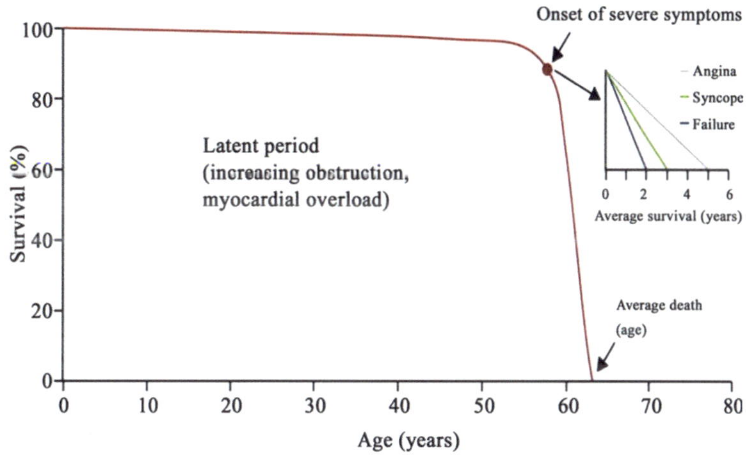

Figure 1.
Natural history of aortic stenosis. A long, latent, asymptomatic period is present followed by a very rapid decline in survival with the onset of symptoms of angina, syncope, and/or heart failure in severe AS patients [8].

and whether elective or early intervention during the asymptomatic stage might be better long term. At present, the surgical mortality for AVR is <2% for severe AS in patients with New York Heart Association (NYHA) functional class I or II heart failure, whereas this risk is significantly higher with class III or IV [13]. Thus, even though the patient may be asymptomatic, AS severity can progress and cause LV dysfunction during the conservative management period and significantly increase the surgical risk [14]. Furthermore, there is concern regarding the development of significant LV myocardial hypertrophy and irreversible myocardial fibrosis due to pressure overload which may result in persistent postoperative diastolic dysfunction and heart failure, even if AVR is successful [15, 16]. However, a general recommendation cannot be made at this time due to insufficient evidence to justify the benefit of AVR in asymptomatic patients to outweigh the risks of surgery and complications related to prosthesis long-term. However, those patients who may benefit from early surgical intervention should be identified through risk stratification [17]. Over the past decade, transcatheter aortic valve replacement (TAVR) has emerged as an alternative treatment strategy for symptomatic severe AS patients who are not suitable or prohibitive for surgical AVR (SAVR) [18, 19] or at high risk for surgery [20, 21]. This technology then expanded to benefit patients with intermediate operative risk, where TAVR using a self-expanding prosthesis was noninferior to SAVR at 24 months follow-up [22]. More recently, TAVR using a balloon-expandable SAPIEN 3 system in low-risk patients was shown to be superior to SAVR based on a composite of death, stroke, and rehospitalization at 1-year follow-up, despite excellent surgical results [23]. Long-term follow-up studies are underway to help determine the true therapeutic impact of TAVR vs. SAVR.

3. Severe AS: definition and rate of hemodynamic progression

AS severity quantitation is based on the degree of LVOT obstruction caused by progressive narrowing of the aortic valve orifice. Echocardiography with Doppler evaluation is the main modality for diagnosing AS. Traditionally, hemodynamic severity of AS has been described based on peak aortic jet velocity (V_{max}), MG, and AVA. According to the 2014 ACC/AHA guidelines, severe AS is defined as $V_{max} \geq 4.0$ m/s, MG ≥ 40 mmHg, and AVA < 1.0 cm^2 [24]. The rate of hemodynamic progression in AS is highly variable. The average rate of progression was reported as increase in V_{max} by 0.3 m/s/year and MG by 7 mmHg/year and decrease in AVA by 0.1 cm^2/year [11]. Studies have shown that the strongest predictors of outcomes in AS were severity of the aortic valve obstruction. During a follow-up period of 2 years, progression of symptoms requiring AVR was about 80% for patients with V_{max} > 4.0 m/s vs. 35% with V_{max} of 3.0–4.0 m/s and 15% for patients with V_{max} < 3.0 m/s. MG and AVA, other parameters of stenosis severity, were also strong predictors of patient outcomes [25].

4. Discrepancies with echocardiographic criteria for grading AS

Echocardiography is the current standard modality for evaluating AS severity. However, challenges due to inconsistencies between measurements of the MG and the calculated AVA in patients with normal systolic function were noted (see **Figure 2**). This finding was attributed primarily to differences in stroke volume and flow across the aortic valve. While it seems possible that discrepancies can occur when the cardiac output is low from reduced LVEF, inconsistent measurements in patients with preserved LVEF were observed. Another potential explanation for the discrepancies was that effective valve area derived by Doppler echocardiography is often smaller than the anatomic valve area measured during cardiac catheterization or by planimetry or at autopsy. So while the initial guidelines for determining AS severity were based on invasive measurements (reflecting the anatomic valve area), echocardiographic Doppler measurements are currently used to make clinical decisions for AS patients still based on the original anatomic valve area criteria. Thus, based on AVA, it is possible that more patients may be categorized as having severe AS

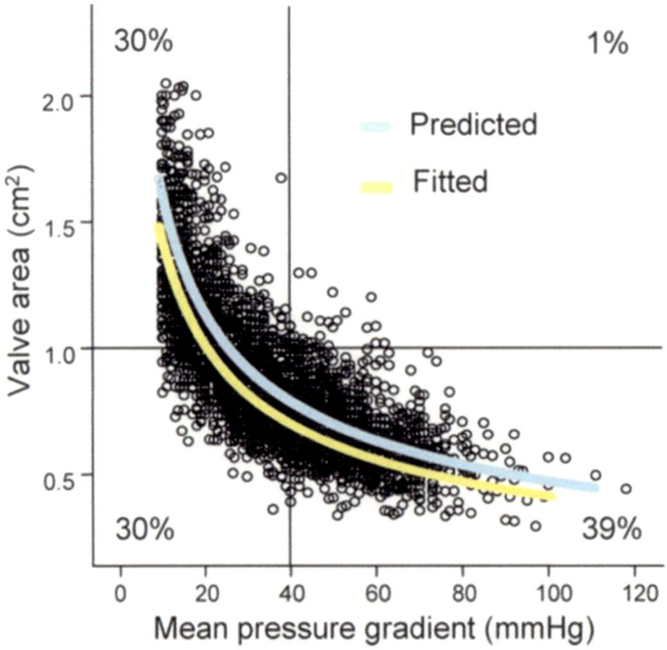

Figure 2.
Comparison of AVA vs. MG in AS patients with preserved LVEF. The predicted values from the Gorlin equation and the fitted curve of the study cohort are shown. The quadrants depict severe AS cutoff points based on the guidelines, and the percentages represent patients per quadrant. Thirty percent of the severe AS patients were diagnosed based on AVA, but not by MG [26].

relative to the peak flow velocity and MG. Therefore, some authors have suggested that AVA cutoff value for severe AS be changed to 0.8 cm^2 [26].

There are other potential etiologies of discrepant AVA and MG measurements in the setting of preserved LVEF which also need to be taken into consideration. First, technical errors need to be excluded. For example, LVOT diameter measurement may be inaccurate, and/or LVOT velocity time integral may be underestimated due to misplacement of the pulsed wave Doppler sample in the LVOT, leading to the underestimation of the stroke volume and the AVA. Second, patients with small body habitus and small LV dimensions could have lower stroke volume and lower transaortic gradient. Therefore, additional diagnostic studies such as dobutamine stress echocardiography (DSE), calcium scoring using multi-detector computed tomography (MDCT), and/or BNP may be necessary to corroborate AS severity and guide management strategy.

5. Hemodynamic classifications of AS

In patients with AVA < 1 cm^2, there are six flow-gradient patterns: NF/VHG, NF/HG, LF/HG, LF/LG with reduced LVEF, LF/LG with preserved LVEF, and NF/LG. VHG is defined as MG ≥ 60 mmHg, and HG is defined as MG ≥ 40 mmHg; stroke volume index (SVI) of normal flow is ≥35 ml/m^2. Low flow is defined as SVI < 35 ml/m^2. Low gradient is defined as MG < 40 mmHg. LF/LG AS with reduced LVEF is present when the gradient is low, the flow is low, and the LVEF is abnormal (<50%). LF/LG AS with preserved LVEF is present when the gradient is low and the flow is low but the LVEF is normal (>50%) (see **Table 1**).

5.1 High-gradient AS

Severe VHG AS ($V_{max} \geq 5.0$ m/s) has significantly worse prognosis than severe HG AS ($V_{max} \geq 4.0$ m/s) [3], so we acknowledge VHG AS as a separate entity from HG AS. However, most studies assessing AS severity using the new classification system combined NF/VHG and NF/HG as one entity under the subgroup of NF/HG. Thus, we will characterize these two groups together and highlight some of the relevant findings for VHG AS.

5.1.1 Normal flow/very high gradient or high gradient

NF/VHG AS pattern is defined as AVA < 1.0 cm^2, MG ≥ 60 mmHg, $V_{max} \geq 5.0$ m/s, and LVEF ≥ 50% with SVI ≥ 35 ml/m^2. NF/HG AS is defined as MG ≥ 40 mmHg and $V_{max} \geq 4$ m/s with the same criteria for AVA, LVEF, and SVI as NF/VHG. Patients with these two flow-gradient patterns are the most prevalent (up to 70%) of all the AS groups. These patients tend to have more severe valvular stenosis suggesting more prolonged exposure to the progressive disease process. Compared with the NF/LG group, there is preservation of LV longitudinal function. However, these patients have higher BNP level and lower cardiac-event free survival [27].

When evaluating AS severity, V_{max} is an important parameter which closely correlates with outcome. One study assessing the outcome of asymptomatic patients with very severe AS found that the higher the velocity, the lower the event-free survival with most patients experiencing some event within 3 years (see **Figure 3**). Patients with $V_{max} \geq 5$ m/s were symptomatic at presentation. Furthermore, asymptomatic patients with $V_{max} \geq 5.5$ m/s were highly likely to develop rapid onset of symptoms [3]. A landmark study evaluating the rate of hemodynamic progression and predictors of outcome in asymptomatic AS patients demonstrated that when V_{max} exceeds 4 m/s, virtually all patients become symptomatic in 5 years.

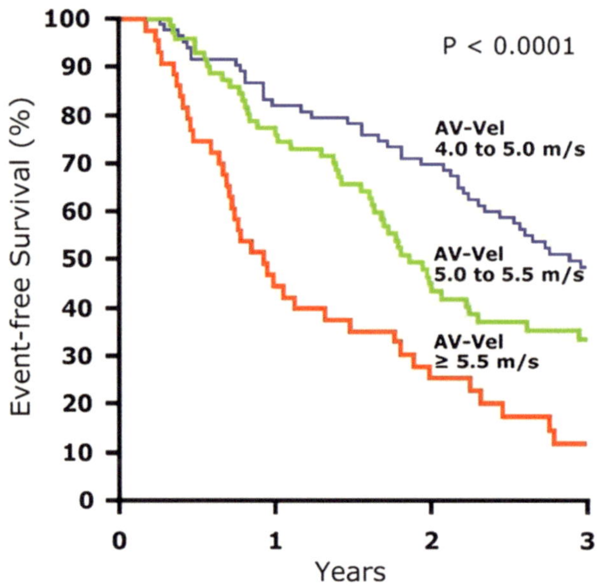

Figure 3.
Event-free survival with very severe AS. Kaplan-Meier estimates demonstrate that maximum aortic jet velocity closely correlates with outcome, with higher the velocity, the lower the event-free survival [3].

The velocity traditionally reflects the chronicity of the degenerative process. V_{max} between 3 and 4 m/s were also found to be not benign, and only 20% of patients remained asymptomatic over 5 years. Only when V_{max} was <3 m/s, there was an 85% chance that the patient will remain asymptomatic for 5 years [11] (see **Figure 4**).

MG is another well-recognized parameter for defining AS severity. One study assessed the prognostic impact of MG on all-cause mortality in severe AS with preserved LVEF. They found that MG > 60 mmHg at baseline was associated with greater risk of all-cause mortality than lower values, thereby justifying a separate hemodynamic classification. The higher MG also reflected the chronicity of the disease process [28] (see **Figure 5**).

AVA < 1.0 cm^2 also correlated with poor outcome compared to moderate or mild categories. More severe AVAs carried worse prognosis, and like V_{max} and MG, they reflected disease chronicity. While the rate of progression is highly variable, the often quoted number is 0.1 cm^2/year [29] (see **Figure 6**). However, when V_{max} was high or very high (4–6 m/s), there was no significant difference in the outcome based on the calculated AVA [3].

According to the current ACC/AHA guidelines, symptomatic NF/HG and NF/VHG severe AS patients have a class I indication for AVR. When asymptomatic, these AS subgroups are recommended to undergo further risk stratification.

5.1.2 Low flow/high gradient

This pattern of AS is defined as AVA < 1.0 cm^2, MG $\geq$ 40 mmHg, and LVEF $\geq$ 50% with SVI < 35 ml/m^2. The prevalence of this AS subtype is much less (8%) [30]. These patients have LV remodeling with reduced longitudinal function despite preserved LVEF. As a consequence, LV output is reduced with resultant lower than expected MG. LF/HG AS patients have shown to have high BNP, and their prognosis is similar or worse than those with NL/HG AS. When symptomatic, these patients have better survival with AVR [27, 31].

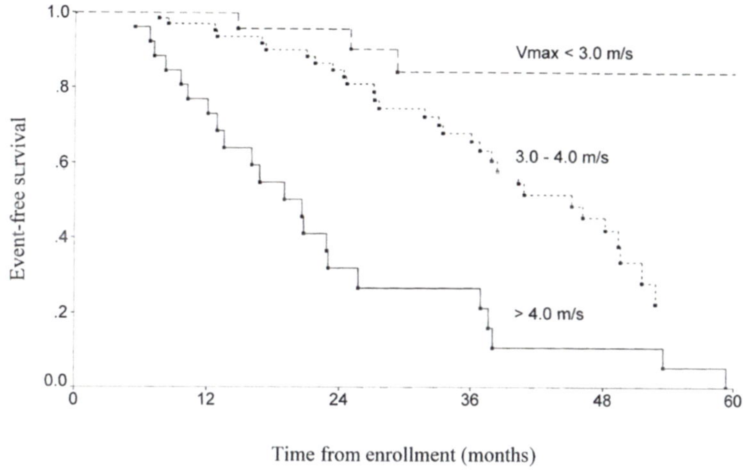

Figure 4.
Effect of V_{max} *on outcomes in asymptomatic AS. Cox regression analysis demonstrating event-free survival in asymptomatic AS patients categorized by initial peak aortic jet velocity [11].*

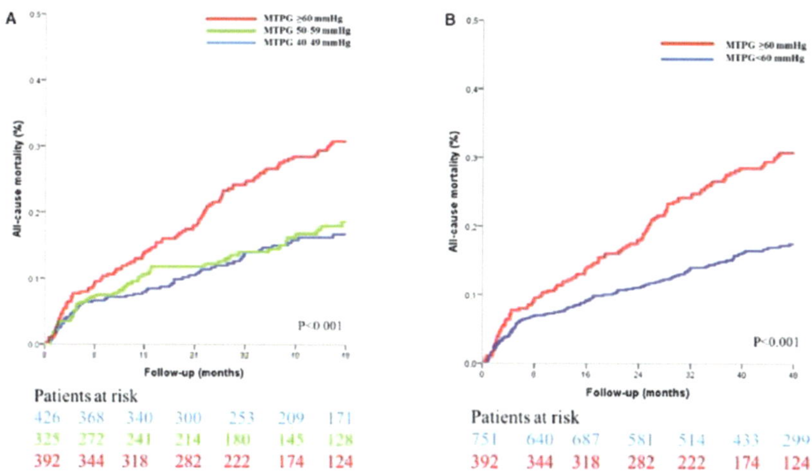

Figure 5.
Impact of MG on outcomes in severe AS. Kaplan-Meier estimates of survival based on MG [28].

5.2 Low-gradient AS

Three types of low-gradient severe AS have been described based on the LVEF and the flow state. LF/LG AS with reduced LVEF (<50%) is present when there is LV systolic dysfunction with reduced stroke volume in the setting of severe AS which results in decreased transvalvular velocity/gradient. If the LVEF is normal (≥50%), the stroke volume index (SVI) helps determine the presence of LF/LG AS with preserved LVEF (if the SVI is low, <35 ml/m^2) or NF/LG AS (if the SVI is normal, ≥35% ml/m^2) [32] (see **Table 2**).

5.2.1 Low flow/low gradient with reduced LVEF

This AS subtype, also known as "classical" LF/LG AS, is defined as AVA < 1.0 cm^2, MG < 40 mmHg, SVI < 35 ml/m^2, and LVEF < 50%. LF/LG AS with

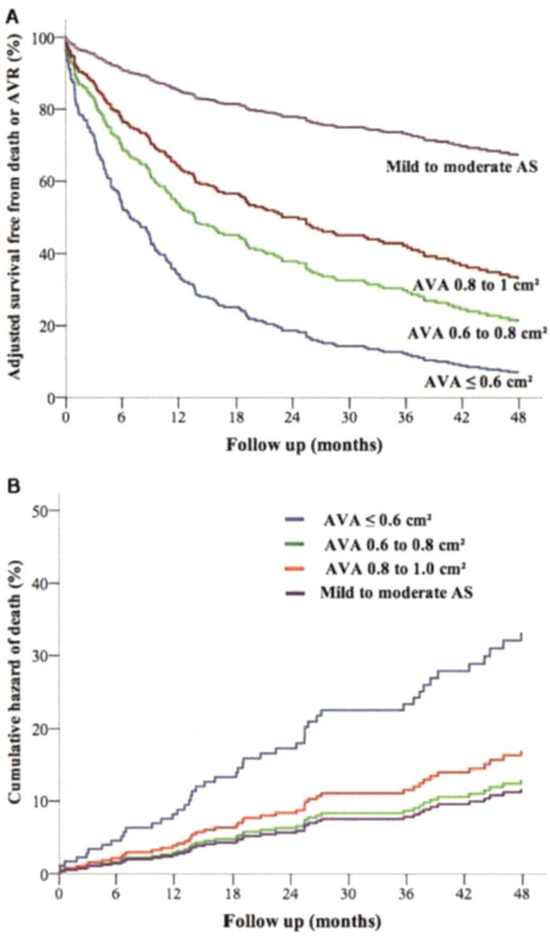

Figure 6.
(A) Adjusted event-free survival based on AVA. (B) Cumulative hazard of death based on AVA [29].

reduced LVEF accounts for about 5–10% of the AS population [33, 34] and has the worst outcome among all the AS categories [30, 33, 34]. The low flow state is usually associated with LV systolic dysfunction either from pressure overload due to the underlying severe AS or cardiomyopathy of another etiology.

In order to differentiate true-severe AS from pseudo-severe AS, low-dose DSE is the initial recommended study to determine whether there is normal flow reserve (an increase in stroke volume of >20%) or diminished flow reserve (see **Figure** 7). Patients with normal flow reserve may have true-severe AS (MG ≥ 40 mmHg with AVA < 1.0 cm^2 at any stage of DSE) which requires AVR or pseudo-severe AS (MG < 40 mmHg with AVA > 1.0 cm^2) where medical therapy is recommended [32, 35]. In patients where the increase in stroke volume with DSE is <20% but >15% and MG is <40 mmHg, the definitive diagnosis of AS severity may remain questionable. In this case, the projected AVA calculation using normal flow rate may be beneficial where a value <1.0 cm^2 is suggestive of true-severe AS [36] (see (Eq. (1)). However, if the stroke volume increase is <15%, further evaluation beyond DSE is often required, and calcium quantification of the aortic valve using MDCT is helpful in confirming the AS severity. The cutoff values for true-severe AS is >1200 AU in women and >2000 AU in men [37, 38].

Valvuloarterial impedance (Zva) is an index to evaluate global LV hemodynamic load using Doppler echocardiography (see Eq. (2)). Zva > 5 has been shown to predict adverse outcomes in patients with AS and LV dysfunction. Since AS is a disease of the elderly, in addition to valvular stenosis, vascular stiffness due to various factors including age and hypertension may be present. As a result, the LV may be subject to a double afterload, known as global LV afterload or Zva. In general, higher Zva is associated with worse outcome. However, since Zva is a flow-dependent parameter, this index may be less reliable in low flow states since small changes in stroke volume can produce large changes in Zva [39].

Low Gradient AS (MG < 40 mmHg, AVA < 1.0 cm2)	**LF/LG AS with reduced LVEF** LVEF < 50%, SVI < 35 ml/m^2
	LF/LG AS with preserved LVEF LVEF ≥ 50%, SVI < 35 ml/m^2
	NF/LG AS LVEF ≥ 50%, SVI ≥ 35 ml/m^2

AS, aortic valve stenosis; MG, mean transaortic gradient; AVA, aortic valve area; LF, low flow; LG, low gradient; NF, normal flow; LVEF, left ventricular ejection fraction; SVI, stroke volume index.

Table 2.
Subclassification of low gradient AS.

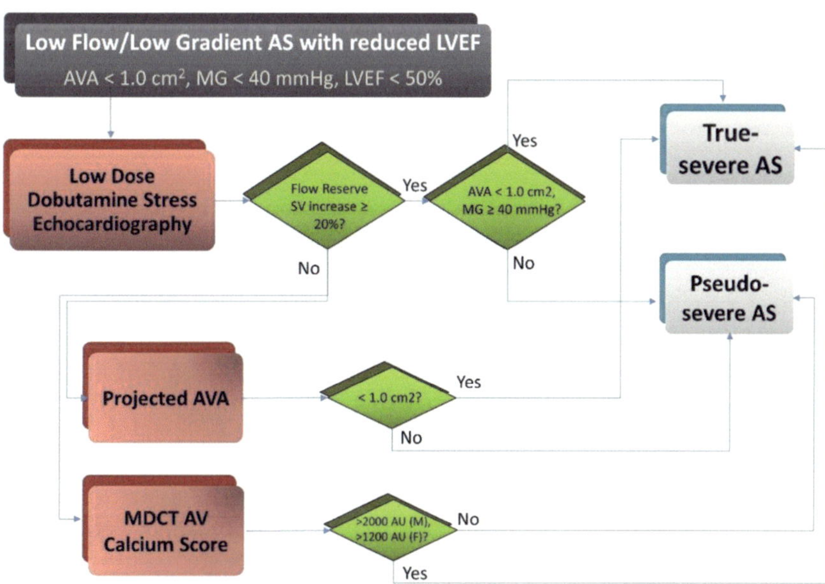

Figure 7.
Algorithm for diagnosing LF/LG AS with reduced LVEF. AS, aortic stenosis; AVA, aortic valve area; MG, mean gradient; LVEF, left ventricular ejection fraction; SV, stroke volume; AV, aortic valve; MDCT, multi-detector computed tomography.

	Recommendation	Class
LF/LG AS with reduced LVEF (Stage D2)	AVR is reasonable in symptomatic patients with low LVEF, LF/LG severe AS with a DSE that shows MG ≥ 40mmHg with AVA < 1.0 cm^2 at any dobutamine dose.	IIa
LF/LG AS with preserved LVEF (Stage D3)	AVR is reasonable in symptomatic patients who have LF/LG severe AS who are normotensive and have an LVEF ≥ 50% if clinical, hemodynamic, and anatomic data support valve obstruction as the most likely cause of symptoms.	IIa

From Nishimura RA, Otto CM, Bonow RO, et al. 2014 AHA/ACC Guideline for the Management of Patients with Valvular Heart Disease: a Report of the American College of Cardiology/American Heart Association Task Force on Practice Guidelines. J Am Coll Cardiol. 2014 Jun 10;63(22):e57-185. AVR, aortic valve replacement, LF, low flow; LG, low gradient; AS, aortic stenosis; LVEF, left ventricular ejection fraction; DSE, dobutamine stress echocardiography; MG, mean gradient, AVA, aortic valve area.

Table 3.
Recommendations for aortic valve replacement in LF/LG AS.

Two-dimensional and three-dimensional transesophageal echocardiography may also be beneficial for confirming AS severity via direct visualization of the aortic valve anatomy and physiology.

In general, LF/LG AS has the worst prognosis compared to the other categories in part because the severity of AS is often under-recognized and surgical treatment is delayed. Patients with LF/LG AS with reduced LVEF have higher adverse event rates and mortality than LF/LG AS with preserved LVEF. The operative risk is also high in this AS subgroup. However, AVR has shown to have significant survival benefit compared to patients undergoing conservative management [40]. Furthermore, TAVR in LF/LG AS with reduced LVEF has demonstrated to have significant survival benefit compared with standard medical therapy in patients who are not suitable for surgery and similar outcomes compared with SAVR for patients at high surgical risk [41]. According to the ACC/AHA guidelines, true-severe LF/LG AS with reduced LVEF has a class IIa indication for AVR [42] (see **Table 3**).

5.2.2 Low flow/low gradient with preserved LVEF

LF/LG AS with preserved LVEF, also described as "paradoxical" LF/LG AS, is defined as AVA < 1.0 cm^2, AVA indexed < 0.6 cm^2/m^2, MG < 40 mmHg, SVI < 35 ml/m^2, and LVEF ≥ 50%. This AS pattern has generated much controversy among investigators. Studies have reported that low flow state is present in about 30% of AS patients with normal LVEF [31, 43–46]. This AS subgroup accounts for about 15–35% of the symptomatic and 5–10% of the asymptomatic AS patients [30]. The classic characteristics described with this AS subtype are small LV cavity size with marked concentric hypertrophy, myocardial fibrosis, restrictive diastolic physiology, reduced LV longitudinal systolic function, and increased global LV afterload resulting in reduced SVI and worse outcome [6, 31, 47]. Other factors associated with this pattern include women, older age, systemic and/or pulmonary hypertension, atrial fibrillation, mitral regurgitation, and right ventricular dysfunction [27, 46]. Some studies have shown that these patients have one of the worst prognoses as the disease severity is often under-recognized and surgery is delayed. This pattern has shown to have better outcomes than LF/LG AS with reduced LVEF but worse outcomes than moderate AS, HG AS, and NF/LG AS [31, 41, 48]. The likelihood of remaining alive in 3 years without AVR has been reported about five fold lower than normal flow state [43].

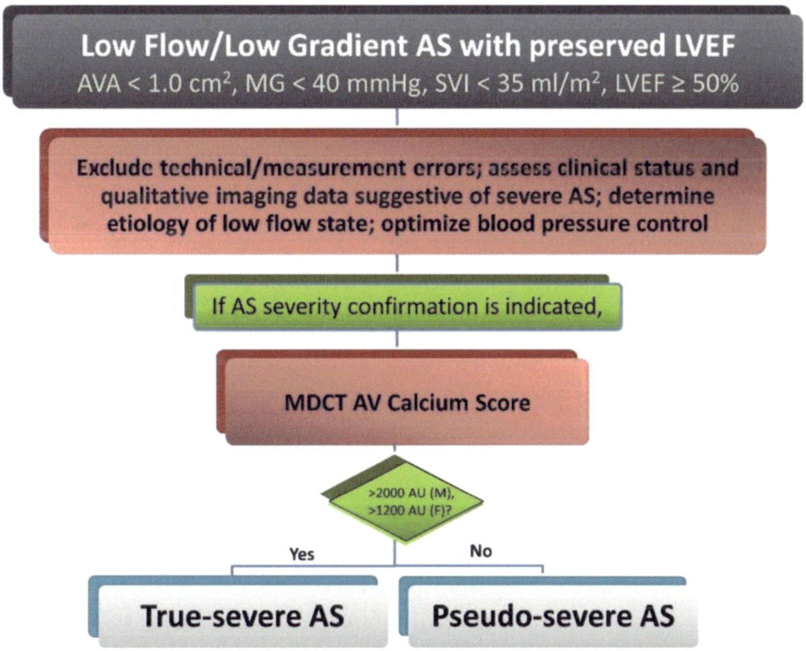

Figure 8.
Algorithm for diagnosing LF/LG AS with preserved LVEF. LF, low flow; LG, low gradient; AS, aortic stenosis; AVA, aortic valve area; MG, mean gradient; LVEF, left ventricular ejection fraction; SVI, stroke volume index; AV, aortic valve; MDCT, multi-detector computed tomography.

When evaluating patients with this AS entity, it is essential to first exclude potential technical errors which may affect the gradient, stroke volume, and AVA measurements. Next, an integrated approach assessing the different criteria to support severe AS needs to be evaluated. These parameters include clinical characteristics such as physical examination suggestive of severe AS, patient symptoms, and the presence of hypertension. Potential etiologies of low flow state need to be considered. Qualitative imaging analyses such as the presence of left ventricular hypertrophy and LV strain measurements should also be assessed. Once LF/LG AS with preserved LVEF status is confirmed, quantitation of aortic valve calcification using MDCT may be helpful in differentiating true-severe vs. pseudo-severe AS [35, 49] (see **Figure 8**). One small study showed that low-dose DSE may be useful in confirming the diagnosis with this entity [50].

According to the ACC/AHA guidelines, LF/LG AS with preserved LVEF has a class IIa indication for AVR, if clinical, anatomic, and hemodynamic data support that the patient's symptom is from the obstructive pathophysiology of the aortic valve [42] (see **Table 3**). One randomized trial data showed significant survival benefit after TAVR compared to standard medical treatment or similar clinical outcomes vs. SAVR [41]. In patients with greater degree of LV myocardial fibrosis, more advanced stage of diastolic dysfunction and low SVI demonstrated worse outcomes after TAVR [51, 52].

In contrast to the findings described above, some other investigators have shown differing results for this AS entity. In one prospective study with a large number of patients with asymptomatic AS, there was no difference between the moderate stenosis and the low-gradient "severe" AS groups in terms of valve-associated events, major cardiovascular events, or cardiac death, even when the groups were subcategorized into low flow and normal flow states [53].

Another large study demonstrated that patients with LF/LG AS with preserved LVEF had better spontaneous survival than the patients with HG severe AS, and the results are unaffected by flow states. Furthermore, the patients with LF/LG AS with preserved LVEF progressed to develop HG AS over time, and in all patients who showed a reduction in transvalvular gradients over time, this decrease was associated with reduction in LVEF [54]. Another study showed that patients with severe LF/LG AS with preserved LVEF had similar outcomes as patients with mild to moderate AS, and there was no significant benefit of AVR in this group [55]. However, a comparison of two studies by Hachicha et al. [31] and Jander et al. [53] showed that there were some differences between the study group findings which may, at least in part, have contributed to the differing outcomes. Some investigators have proposed for reducing the AVA cutoff value for severe AS closer to $\leq 0.8\ cm^2$ to avoid overestimation of AS severity [56].

5.2.3 Normal flow/low gradient

This AS pattern is defined as AVA < $1.0\ cm^2$, AVA indexed < $0.6\ cm^2$, MG < 40 mmHg, and LVEF ≥ 50% with SVI ≥ $35\ ml/m^2$. NF/LG AS has shown to be present in about one third of AS patients [30], and some studies have suggested that this AS pattern may be due to marked reduction in transaortic gradient from systemic hypertension and decreased aortic compliance [57, 58]. Patients with NL/LG AS are reported to have less severe disease than the other AS categories with lower BNP and preserved LV longitudinal function [35]. In terms of diagnosis, technical measurement errors need to be excluded, and aortic valve calcium scoring using MDCT may be beneficial to further determine the AS severity [38]. According to the 2017 European Association of Cardiovascular Imaging and the American Society of Echocardiography Recommendations, however, this entity is considered to be due to measurement errors or the consequence of inconsistent cutoff values for transaortic velocity/gradient and AVA [35]. Some studies have supported this thought as patients in the NF/LG AS subgroup demonstrated the same outcome as patients with moderate AS [59].

There are no particular recommendations for this subgroup in the current guidelines, and AVR should only be considered in symptomatic patients with confirmed severe AS. One study showed survival benefit in these patients [43], while another study showed no difference in survival in patients who underwent early AVR compared to conservative management [60].

Projected AVA calculation

$$\text{Projected AVA} = \text{AVArest} + \left(\frac{\Delta\,\text{AVA}}{\Delta\,\boldsymbol{Q}}\right) * (\mathbf{250} - \boldsymbol{Q}\text{rest})$$

$$\Delta\,\text{AVA} = \text{AVApeak} - \text{AVArest} \;=\; \text{Change in AVA at rest and at peak DSE}$$

$$\Delta\,\text{Q} = \text{Qpeak} - \text{Qrest} \;=\; \text{Change in } \boldsymbol{Q} \text{ at rest and at peak DSE} \tag{1}$$

Projected AVA at a normal flow rate (250 ml/s) <$1.0\ cm^2$ suggests severe AS.

AVArest, aortic valve area at rest; DSE, dobutamine stress echocardiography; AVApeak, aortic valve area at peak; Qrest, stroke volume at rest; Qpeak, stroke volume at peak DSE.

Valvuloarterial impedance calculation

$$Zva = \frac{\text{Systemic Arterial Pressure} + \text{Mean Pressure Gradient}}{\text{Stroke Volume Index}}$$

$$Zva = \text{Valvuloarterial Impedence} \tag{2}$$

6. Conclusions

The different hemodynamic categories of severe AS have shown to have varying clinical outcomes. Low flow state has exhibited the worst prognosis due to intrinsic myocardial dysfunction and/or under-recognition of the disease severity resulting in inappropriate delay in AVR. Low-gradient AS with low flow state is of particular challenge for clinical decision-making, especially when differentiating true-severe AS (where AVR may be beneficial) vs. pseudo-severe AS (where conservative medical management is appropriate). In LF/LG AS with reduced LVEF, DSE is beneficial for the confirmation of AS severity and risk stratification. In the setting of partial or no flow reserve, projected AVA and/or calcium scoring with MDCT may be useful to guide management. LF/LG AS with preserved LVEF is an entity where the natural history and the pathophysiology are not well understood. There has been much controversy and differing schools of thought around this AS subgroup. Numerous studies have shown that LF/LG AS with preserved LVEF is associated with poor prognosis, and therefore, careful evaluation and identification of these patients are necessary to ensure proper management. Calcium quantification using MDCT has shown to be the preferred technique for confirming AS severity with this subgroup. However, other investigators have reported that this AS entity represents moderate AS with no significant difference in outcomes between the groups. These discrepant findings may be resolved based on more randomized studies with large cohorts and with the application of more advanced diagnostic imaging techniques capable of overcoming the limitations of the currently available technology to better assess AS severity. In symptomatic high-gradient severe AS, regardless of the flow state, AVR is the only treatment option that has demonstrated to improve symptoms and survival. In asymptomatic high-gradient severe AS, regardless of the flow state, the current guidelines recommend watchful waiting and conservative management, although controversy exists about the optimal timing of intervention.

Over the years, the operative risk for SAVR for severe AS has significantly decreased, and TAVR has emerged as a promising alternative treatment for these patients with different operative risk profiles—high, intermediate, and more recently low risk. Recent data have supported that TAVR is superior or noninferior to SAVR in the treatment of severe AS and long-term follow-up assessment will better validate the true comparison between the two approaches and determine the optimal treatment strategy. As the TAVR technology continues to advance, the next generations of bioprostheses will be introduced which may further improve outcomes. Therefore, it is vital to accurately diagnose AS severity and identify those individuals who may benefit from AVR in a timely manner to optimize patient care and clinical outcomes.

Conflict of interest

None.

Author details

Susan Kwon and Aasha Gopal*
St. Francis Hospital, Roslyn, New York, USA

*Address all correspondence to: aasha.gopal@gmail.com

References

[1] Nkomo VT et al. Burden of valvular heart diseases: A population-based study. Lancet. 2006;**368**(9540):1005-1011

[2] Otto CM, Prendergast B. Aortic-valve stenosis—From patients at risk to severe valve obstruction. The New England Journal of Medicine. 2014;**371**(8):744-756

[3] Rosenhek R et al. Natural history of very severe aortic stenosis. Circulation. 2010;**121**(1):151-156

[4] Pai RG et al. Malignant natural history of asymptomatic severe aortic stenosis: Benefit of aortic valve replacement. The Annals of Thoracic Surgery. 2006;**82**(6):2116-2122

[5] Nishimura RA et al. 2014 AHA/ACC guideline for the management of patients with valvular heart disease: Executive summary: A report of the American College of Cardiology/American Heart Association Task Force on Practice Guidelines. Journal of the American College of Cardiology. 2014;**63**(22):2438-2488

[6] Dumesnil JG, Pibarot P, Carabello B. Paradoxical low flow and/or low gradient severe aortic stenosis despite preserved left ventricular ejection fraction: Implications for diagnosis and treatment. European Heart Journal. 2010;**31**(3):281-289

[7] Rosenhek R et al. Predictors of outcome in severe, asymptomatic aortic stenosis. The New England Journal of Medicine. 2000;**343**(9):611-617

[8] Ross J Jr, Braunwald E. Aortic stenosis. Circulation. 1968;**38**(1 Suppl):61-67

[9] Braunwald E. On the natural history of severe aortic stenosis. Journal of the American College of Cardiology. 1990;**15**(5):1018-1020

[10] Nessmith MG et al. Usefulness of an elevated B-type natriuretic peptide in predicting survival in patients with aortic stenosis treated without surgery. The American Journal of Cardiology. 2005;**96**(10):1445-1448

[11] Otto CM et al. Prospective study of asymptomatic valvular aortic stenosis. Clinical, echocardiographic, and exercise predictors of outcome. Circulation. 1997;**95**(9):2262-2270

[12] Pellikka PA et al. The natural history of adults with asymptomatic, hemodynamically significant aortic stenosis. Journal of the American College of Cardiology. 1990;**15**(5):1012-1017

[13] Pierard S et al. Impact of preoperative symptoms on postoperative survival in severe aortic stenosis: Implications for the timing of surgery. The Annals of Thoracic Surgery. 2014;**97**(3):803-809

[14] Halkos ME et al. Aortic valve replacement for aortic stenosis in patients with left ventricular dysfunction. The Annals of Thoracic Surgery. 2009;**88**(3):746-751

[15] Azevedo CF et al. Prognostic significance of myocardial fibrosis quantification by histopathology and magnetic resonance imaging in patients with severe aortic valve disease. Journal of the American College of Cardiology. 2010;**56**(4):278-287

[16] Weidemann F et al. Impact of myocardial fibrosis in patients with symptomatic severe aortic stenosis. Circulation. 2009;**120**(7):577-584

[17] Rosenhek R, Maurer G, Baumgartner H. Should early elective surgery be performed in patients with severe but asymptomatic aortic stenosis? European Heart Journal. 2002;**23**(18):1417-1421

[18] Leon MB et al. Transcatheter aortic-valve implantation for aortic stenosis in patients who cannot undergo surgery. The New England Journal of Medicine. 2010;**363**(17):1597-1607

[19] Popma JJ et al. Transcatheter aortic valve replacement using a self-expanding bioprosthesis in patients with severe aortic stenosis at extreme risk for surgery. Journal of the American College of Cardiology. 2014;**63**(19):1972-1981

[20] Smith CR et al. Transcatheter versus surgical aortic-valve replacement in high-risk patients. The New England Journal of Medicine. 2011;**364**(23):2187-2198

[21] Adams DH, Popma JJ, Reardon MJ. Transcatheter aortic-valve replacement with a self-expanding prosthesis. The New England Journal of Medicine. 2014;**371**(10):967-968

[22] Reardon MJ et al. Surgical or transcatheter aortic-valve replacement in intermediate-risk patients. The New England Journal of Medicine. 2017;**376**(14):1321-1331

[23] Mack MJ et al. Transcatheter aortic-valve replacement with a balloon-expandable valve in low-risk patients. The New England Journal of Medicine. 2 May 2019;**380**(18):1695-1705

[24] Nishimura RA et al. 2014 AHA/ACC guideline for the management of patients with valvular heart disease: A report of the American College of Cardiology/American Heart Association Task Force on Practice Guidelines. Circulation. 2014;**129**(23):e521-e643

[25] Vahanian A, Otto CM. Risk stratification of patients with aortic stenosis. European Heart Journal. 2010;**31**(4):416-423

[26] Minners J et al. Inconsistencies of echocardiographic criteria for the grading of aortic valve stenosis. European Heart Journal. 2008;**29**(8):1043-1048

[27] Lancellotti P, Davin L, Dulgheru R. Aortic stenosis grading and outcome: New categories, new therapeutic challenges. JACC: Cardiovascular Imaging. 2016;**9**(11):1264-1266

[28] Bohbot Y et al. Impact of mean transaortic pressure gradient on long-term outcome in patients with severe aortic stenosis and preserved left ventricular ejection fraction. Journal of the American Heart Association. 2017;**6**(6):e005850. DOI: 10.1161/JAHA 117.005850

[29] Marechaux S et al. Prognostic value of aortic valve area by Doppler echocardiography in patients with severe asymptomatic aortic stenosis. Journal of the American Heart Association. 2016;**5**(5):e003146. DOI: 10.1161/JAHA. 115.003146

[30] Lancellotti P. Grading aortic stenosis severity when the flow modifies the gradientvalve area correlation. Cardiovascular Diagnosis and Therapy. 2012;**2**(1):6-9

[31] Hachicha Z et al. Paradoxical low-flow, low-gradient severe aortic stenosis despite preserved ejection fraction is associated with higher afterload and reduced survival. Circulation. 2007;**115**(22):2856-2864

[32] Pibarot P, Dumesnil JG. Low-flow, low-gradient aortic stenosis with normal and depressed left ventricular ejection fraction. Journal of the American College of Cardiology. 2012;**60**(19):1845-1853

[33] Connolly HM et al. Aortic valve replacement for aortic stenosis with severe left ventricular dysfunction. Prognostic indicators. Circulation. 1997;**95**(10):2395-2400

[34] Connolly HM et al. Severe aortic stenosis with low transvalvular

gradient and severe left ventricular dysfunction: Result of aortic valve replacement in 52 patients. Circulation. 2000;**101**(16):1940-1946

[35] Baumgartner HC et al. Recommendations on the echocardiographic assessment of aortic valve stenosis: A focused update from the European Association of Cardiovascular Imaging and the American Society of Echocardiography. European Heart Journal Cardiovascular Imaging. 2017;**18**(3):254-275

[36] Clavel MA et al. Validation of conventional and simplified methods to calculate projected valve area at normal flow rate in patients with low flow, low gradient aortic stenosis: The multicenter TOPAS (True or Pseudo Severe Aortic Stenosis) study. Journal of the American Society of Echocardiography. 2010;**23**(4):380-386

[37] Cueff C et al. Measurement of aortic valve calcification using multislice computed tomography: Correlation with haemodynamic severity of aortic stenosis and clinical implication for patients with low ejection fraction. Heart. 2011;**97**(9):721-726

[38] Clavel MA et al. The complex nature of discordant severe calcified aortic valve disease grading: New insights from combined Doppler echocardiographic and computed tomographic study. Journal of the American College of Cardiology. 2013;**62**(24):2329-2338

[39] Lancellotti P, Magne J. Valvuloarterial impedance in aortic stenosis: Look at the load, but do not forget the flow. European Journal of Echocardiography. 2011;**12**(5):354-357

[40] Tribouilloy C et al. Outcome after aortic valve replacement for low-flow/low-gradient aortic stenosis without contractile reserve on dobutamine stress echocardiography. Journal of the American College of Cardiology. 2009;**53**(20):1865-1873

[41] Herrmann HC et al. Predictors of mortality and outcomes of therapy in low-flow severe aortic stenosis: A Placement of Aortic transcatheter Valves (PARTNER) trial analysis. Circulation. 2013;**127**(23):2316-2326

[42] Nishimura RA et al. 2014 AHA/ACC guideline for the management of patients with valvular heart disease: A report of the American College of Cardiology/American Heart Association Task Force on Practice Guidelines. Journal of the American College of Cardiology. 2014;**63**(22):e57-e185

[43] Lancellotti P et al. Clinical outcome in asymptomatic severe aortic stenosis: Insights from the new proposed aortic stenosis grading classification. Journal of the American College of Cardiology. 2012;**59**(3):235-243

[44] Mohty D et al. Outcome and impact of surgery in paradoxical low-flow, low-gradient severe aortic stenosis and preserved left ventricular ejection fraction: A cardiac catheterization study. Circulation. 2013;**128** (11 Suppl 1):S235-S242

[45] Ozkan A et al. Impact of aortic valve replacement on outcome of symptomatic patients with severe aortic stenosis with low gradient and preserved left ventricular ejection fraction. Circulation. 2013;**128**(6):622-631

[46] Eleid MF et al. Flow-gradient patterns in severe aortic stenosis with preserved ejection fraction: Clinical characteristics and predictors of survival. Circulation. 2013;**128**(16):1781-1789

[47] Adda J et al. Low-flow, low-gradient severe aortic stenosis despite normal ejection fraction is associated with severe left ventricular dysfunction

as assessed by speckle-tracking echocardiography: A multicenter study. Circulation. Cardiovascular Imaging. 2012;**5**(1):27-35

[48] Clavel MA et al. Outcome of patients with aortic stenosis, small valve area, and low-flow, low-gradient despite preserved left ventricular ejection fraction. Journal of the American College of Cardiology. 2012;**60**(14):1259-1267

[49] Clavel MA, Magne J, Pibarot P. Low-gradient aortic stenosis. European Heart Journal. 2016;**37**(34):2645-2657

[50] Clavel MA et al. Stress echocardiography to assess stenosis severity and predict outcome in patients with paradoxical low-flow, low-gradient aortic stenosis and preserved LVEF. JACC: Cardiovascular Imaging. 2013;**6**(2):175-183

[51] Le Ven F et al. Impact of low flow on the outcome of high-risk patients undergoing transcatheter aortic valve replacement. Journal of the American College of Cardiology. 2013;**62**(9):782-788

[52] Herrmann S et al. Low-gradient aortic valve stenosis myocardial fibrosis and its influence on function and outcome. Journal of the American College of Cardiology. 2011;**58**(4):402-412

[53] Jander N et al. Outcome of patients with low-gradient "severe" aortic stenosis and preserved ejection fraction. Circulation. 2011;**123**(8):887-895

[54] Maes F et al. Natural history of paradoxical low-gradient severe aortic stenosis. Circulation. Cardiovascular Imaging. 2014;**7**(4):714-722

[55] Tribouilloy C et al. Low-gradient, low-flow severe aortic stenosis with preserved left ventricular ejection fraction: Characteristics, outcome, and implications for surgery. Journal of the American College of Cardiology. 2015;**65**(1):55-66

[56] Zoghbi WA. Low-gradient "severe" aortic stenosis with normal systolic function: Time to refine the guidelines? Circulation. 2011;**123**(8):838-840

[57] Eleid MF et al. Systemic hypertension in low-gradient severe aortic stenosis with preserved ejection fraction. Circulation. 2013;**128**(12):1349-1353

[58] Kadem L et al. Impact of systemic hypertension on the assessment of aortic stenosis. Heart. 2005;**91**(3):354-361

[59] Mehrotra P et al. Differential left ventricular remodelling and longitudinal function distinguishes low flow from normal-flow preserved ejection fraction low-gradient severe aortic stenosis. European Heart Journal. 2013;**34**(25):1906-1914

[60] Kang DH et al. Watchful observation versus early aortic valve replacement for symptomatic patients with normal flow, low-gradient severe aortic stenosis. Heart. 2015;**101**(17):1375-1381